TOPICS IN
CLINICAL UROLOGY

MEDICAL AND SURGICAL MANAGEMENT OF PROSTATE CANCER

TOPICS IN CLINICAL UROLOGY

Series Editors
Martin I. Resnick, M.D.
Jack S. Elder, M.D.

New Techniques in Reconstructive Urology
Jack W. McAninch, M.D.

Complications of Interventional Techniques
Culley C. Carson III, M.D.

Pediatric Urology for the General Urologist
Jack S. Elder, M.D.

New Developments in the Management of Urolithiasis
James E. Lingeman, M.D.
Glenn M. Preminger, M.D.

New Diagnostic Tests
Martin I. Resnick, M.D.
J. Patrick Spirnak, M.D.

Medical and Surgical Management of Prostate Cancer
Richard G. Middleton, M.D.

Techniques for Ablation of Benign and Malignant Prostate Tissue
Joseph A. Smith, Jr., M.D.
Douglas F. Milam, M.D.

Evaluation and Treatment of Urinary Incontinence
Jerry G. Blaivas, M.D.

TOPICS IN CLINICAL UROLOGY

MEDICAL AND SURGICAL MANAGEMENT OF PROSTATE CANCER

Richard G. Middleton, M.D.
Chairman, Division of Urology
University of Utah
School of Medicine
Salt Lake City, Utah

IGAKU-SHOIN NEW YORK • TOKYO

Published and distributed by

IGAKU-SHOIN Medical Publishers, Inc.
One Madison Avenue, New York, New York 10010

IGAKU-SHOIN Ltd.,
5-24-3 Hongo, Bunkyo-ku, Tokyo 113-91.

Library of Congress Cataloging-in-Publication Data

Medical and surgical management of prostate cancer / [edited by]
Richard G. Middleton, Jr.
p. cm. — (Topics in clinical urology)
Includes bibliographical references and index.
1. Prostate—Cancer. 2. Prostate—Cancer—Surgery. I. Series.
[DNLM: 1. Prostatic Neoplasms—therapy. WJ 752 M488 1996]
RC280.P7M426 1996
616.99′463—dc20
DNLM/DLC
for Library of Congress 95-52984
CIP

ISBN: 0-89640-293-2 (New York)
ISBN: 4-260-14293-3 (Tokyo)

Printed and bound in the U.S.A.
10 9 8 7 6 5 4 3 2 1

PREFACE

The medical literature relating to prostate cancer is extensive, and even when one attempts to review reported experiences with the treatment of prostate cancer, the medical literature is enormous and contains conflicting data and varying therapeutic recommendations. The AUA Guidelines Committee for Prostate Cancer spent five years reviewing reported outcomes with various treatments for stage B adenocarcinoma of the prostate. The committee concluded that it is impossible to compare outcomes of radical prostatectomy, external beam radiation and surveillance in cases of localized prostate cancer. Patient groups subjected to these forms of management have been too dissimilar, and the methods of reporting outcome data have been far from uniform.

The purpose of this volume is not to attempt to review the world's literature, but to focus upon common problems faced by urologists and oncologists in dealing with individual patients with prostate cancer. The articles are addressed to those who specialize in prostate cancer treatment, as well as to residents and fellows in the fields of urology, medical and radiation oncology.

Approaches to various stages of prostate cancer are reviewed and discussed. Experiences with surgery, external beam radiation therapy, and surveillance, as well as cryotherapy, are reported. The selection of appropriate candidates for these various therapies is examined. Modifications of the radical prostatectomy are presented and discussed. Management methods for surgical complications are reviewed. Post prostatectomy incontinence and impotence are discussed and there are chapters on the treatment of rectal injury and alternative treatments for biochemical failure (rising PSA) after radical prostatectomy.

This volume does not address all management problems in dealing with prostate cancer, but some of the most common controversial areas are discussed by selected experts with considerable experience in prostate cancer management.

As editor, I am indebted to the authors for their time, energy expended, and for their experience and wisdom reflected in their contributions to this volume.

Richard G. Middleton, M.D.

CONTRIBUTORS

Peter R. Carroll, M.D.
University of California at San Francisco
Department of Urology
San Francisco, California

John A. Connolly
Department of Urology
University of California School of Medicine
San Francisco, California
The Program in Urologic Oncology, UCSF/Mt. Zion Cancer Center and San Francisco Veterans Administration Medical Center

Gregg R. Eure, M.D.
Assistant Professor
Department of Urology
Virginia Prostate Center
Eastern Virginia Medical School
Sentara Cancer Institute
Norfolk, Virginia

Robert C. Flanigan, M.D.
Department of Urology
Loyola University Medical Center
Maywood, Illinois

Richard F. Labasky, M.D.
Division of Urology
University of Utah
School of Medicine
Salt Lake City, Utah

Paul H. Lange, M.D.
Professor and Chairman
Department of Urology
University of Washington
Seattle, Washington

Bruce A. Lowe, M.D.
Associate Professor of Urology
Oregon Health Sciences University
Portland, Oregon

Sean P. Manion, M.D.
Department of Urology
Loyola University Medical Center
Maywood, Illinois

Richard G. Middleton, M.D.
Chairman, Division of Urology
University of Utah
School of Medicine
Salt Lake City, Utah

James E. Montie, M.D.
Section of Urology
University of Michigan
School of Medicine
Ann Arbor, Michigan

Joseph C. Presti, Jr.
Department of Urology
University of California School of Medicine
San Francisco, California
The Program in Urologic Oncology, UCSF/Mt. Zion Cancer Center and San Francisco Veterans Administration Medical Center

Thomas A. Rozanski, M.D.
Urology Service
Brooke Army Medical Center
San Antonio, Texas

Richard A. Santucci, M.D.
Resident, Department of Urology
University of Washington
Seattle, Washington

Paul F. Schellhammer, M.D.
Professor and Chairman
Department of Urology
Virginia Prostate Center
Eastern Virginia Medical School
Sentara Cancer Institute
Norfolk, Virginia

Katsuto Shinohara
Department of Urology
University of California School of Medicine
San Francisco, California
The Program in Urologic Oncology,
UCSF/Mt. Zion Cancer Center and San Francisco Veterans Administration Medical Center

William U. Shipley, M.D.
Professor, Department of Radiation Oncology
Massachusetts General Hospital
Harvard Medical School
Boston, Massachusetts

Joseph A. Smith, Jr., M.D.
William L. Bray Professor and Chairman
Vanderbilt University Medical Center
Department of Urology
Nashville, Tennessee

Robert A. Stephenson, M.D.
Division of Urology
Department of Surgery
University of Utah
School of Medicine
Salt Lake City, Utah

Ian M. Thompson, M.D.
Chief, Urology Service
Brooke Army Medical Center
San Antonio, Texas

Martha K. Tibbs, M.D.
Resident, Department of Radiation Oncology
Massachusetts General Hospital
Harvard Medical School
Boston, Massachusetts

Anthony L. Zietman, M.D.
Assistant Professor, Department of Radiation Oncology
Massachusetts General Hospital
Harvard Medical School
Boston, Massachusetts

CONTENTS

TOPICS IN
CLINICAL UROLOGY

MEDICAL AND SURGICAL MANAGEMENT OF PROSTATE CANCER

1

Selection of Patients for Radical Prostatectomy

Joseph A. Smith, Jr.

Some men who are subjected to radical prostatectomy for carcinoma of the prostate do not need the operation because they have a tumor never destined to become clinically significant in their lifetime. Others die from prostate cancer despite having undergone surgery with curative intent. However, another group of men who have a radical prostatectomy are cured of a cancer which otherwise would have been a cause of premature mortality. The key issue facing a clinician is how to identify before surgery patients most likely to fall into these categories and to exclude from surgery those unlikely to derive a meaningful benefit. Thus, appropriate selection of patients for radical prostatectomy remains one of the major challenges facing urologic surgeons.

WHEN IS CANCER CLINICALLY SIGNIFICANT?

Other than, perhaps, the psychological effect of knowing that their cancer has been treated adequately, patients with prostate cancer never destined to be of clinical significance derive no meaningful benefit from radical prostatectomy. Statistics alone indicate that the sizeable majority of men with a histologic diagnosis of prostate cancer have tumors which are not life threatening even if left untreated.[1] The argument that surgery benefits a large number of men by eliminating the bone pain and other features of the disease which may occur at an advanced stage even if a man is not destined to die from the disease seems specious. The overwhelming majority of men who suffer these complications are also those who die from the disease. Stated simply, men who benefit from radical prostatectomy are those who otherwise would have died from prostate cancer but do not because of surgery.

A number of factors enter into a projection of the clinical significance of a particular prostate cancer. Unfortunately, none are of sufficient prognostic value to allow accurate prediction in an individual man. However, it is worthwhile to consider these various factors as they are strongly influential in selecting patients for radical prostatectomy.

Patient Factors

Radical prostatectomy should not be performed to prevent men from dying from prostate cancer within 5 years of surgery. This is not to say that rapid disease progression and death from disease may not occur within a relatively short time after diagnosis of apparently localized disease. However, cancers that fall into this category are understaged clinically and are not curable by radical prostatectomy (or any other treatment) anyway. Certainly, the median time to progression to metastatic cancer from a localized disease state in men with carcinoma of the prostate is greater than 5 years and, in many, longer than 10 years. Therefore, it is generally accepted that men should not undergo radical prostatectomy unless they otherwise have a projected longevity of at least 10 years.

A number of factors are used to predict remaining life years including age, family history, and comorbid conditions. However, just as there is variability in predicting the rate of progression of a particular cancer, extreme variability exists in projecting duration of survival for any individual.

Chronologic age is an important criterion but, obviously, should only be viewed in relative terms and in the context of overall medical condition. Nonetheless, statistics on longevity simply do not support the role of radical prostatectomy in men over the age of 75 years with, perhaps, rare exceptions. On the other hand, life insurance actuarial tables and other sources show that a man of less than 70 years of age in good health has an average of 10 or more years of life remaining.

Tumor Volume

If cancer growth can be considered a continuum from preneoplastic changes to metastasis and death of the host, tumor volume can be a surrogate predictor of the intercept point on the cancer growth time-line. From this perspective, tumors of low volume have a longer time to grow until they metastasize than those of larger size at the time of discovery.[2]

For many patients, this concept seems valid. However, the reality is much more complex. The histologic presence of prostate cancer in autopsy series vastly exceeds the clinical rate of the disease. Furthermore, it appears that many of these "autopsy" cancers are not simply in a preclinical growth phase. The average tumor volume in cancers detected at the time of autopsy is less than 0.2 cc.[3] There is no consensus of opinion on the volume at which a tumor should be considered clinically significant, but the vast majority of cancers diagnosed by current methods of detection exceed 0.2 cc in volume.[4]

Retrospective studies after radical prostatectomy which examine tumor volume are instructive.[5] However, the day-to-day clinical issue is how to predict volume preoperatively. Digital rectal examination is notoriously poor at determining tumor volume. Furthermore, increasing numbers of patients in contemporary clinical series have nonpalpable tumors.

Transrectal ultrasound (TRUS) is the most widely used imaging modality for the prostate. Although there is some variability, ultrasound is probably the best method for determining overall prostate volume.[6] Many prostate cancers can be imaged by TRUS, including some nonpalpable tumors. However, definition of the margin of tumors is difficult and imprecise. Furthermore, the typical tumor configuration does not lend itself to geometric calculations.

In many clinical series, stage T1c cancers comprise the majority of men undergoing radical prostatectomy. Since, by definition, these tumors are nonpalpable and detected because of an abnormality in prostate specific antigen (PSA), how can the volume of tumor be determined? Concerns have been expressed that PSA driven prostate biopsies detect large numbers of clinically insignificant cancers.[7] Is there not a chance that random needle biopsy sampling of the prostate will show cancer based upon the prevalence of histologic disease?

We reported histologic findings in 142 men undergoing radical prostatectomy for T1c cancers.[8] One patient had no identifiable tumor in the specimen and a small percentage had scattered foci of microscopic disease (Table 1.1). Presumably, these men were not at risk from their cancer unless the duration of exposure was exceedingly long. Almost one-fourth of men had tumors which were more than microscopic foci but had a volume of less than 1 cc. These are not equivalent to autopsy cancers but they surely were diagnosed early. The important observation is that almost three-fourths of the men had cancers that exceeded 1 cc in size. By almost any volume criteria, these tumors would be considered clinically significant in a man with at least 10 years of life expectancy otherwise.[2]

TABLE 1.1. Relationship of PSA Levels to Tumor Grade, Volume and Pathologic Findings in 142 Patients Undergoing Radical Prostatectomy for Stage T1c Prostate Cancer at Vanderbilt University

	PSA (ng/ml)			
	4 to 9.9	*10 to 14.9*	*15 to 20*	*Totals*
Gleason sum				
2 to 4	17	3	1	21
5 to 7	80	24	6	110
8 to 10	5	3	3	11
	102	30	10	142
Tumor volume				
None	1	—	—	1
Microscopic only	7	—	1	8
Less than 1 cc	33	6	1	40
More than 1 cc	60	25	8	93
Totals	101	31	10	142
Pathologic findings				
Number of patients	102	30	10	142
Capsular penetration	17	10	1	28
Extracapsular extension	31	9	3	43
Seminal vesicle invasion	4	3	2	10
Positive margin	24	10	3	37

Sextant biopsies of the prostate do not seem to be capable of "hitting" an autopsy type of cancer because of random sampling alone.[9] Indiscriminate biopsy of the prostate in men without palpable or biochemical suggestion of disease rarely yields a histologic diagnosis of cancer.[10] In an investigation of familial influences, we performed prostate biopsy on the brothers of men with a diagnosis of the disease and found cancer in 27%.[11] As a "control" group, we also biopsied the brothers-in-law. Although autopsy studies tell us that significant numbers of these brothers-in-law had histologic cancer within the prostate, none had a biopsy that was positive. Although considerations about clinical significance in a particular patient are valid and imperative, a needle biopsy of the prostate that shows cancer despite a prostate gland that is normal to palpation should not be dismissed lightly. Autopsy cancers are rarely included in the category of clinical T1c prostate cancer.

Tumor Grade

When tumors are of low volume, they usually are low-grade. As the size increases, the tumor takes on a less differentiated appearance. Tumor grade alone, then, is a highly predictive criterion. The clinical significance of higher grade tumors is rarely in question. More to the point is whether these lesions are curable given the likelihood of positive margins, if not subclinical metastatic disease.

Despite the concern that high-grade tumors frequently have a poor outcome, a high Gleason grade alone should not exclude a patient from radical prostatectomy. Low-volume, intracapsular yet high-grade lesions clearly exist. Thus, tumor grade is an important yet single criterion in determining clinical significance and curability of apparently localized prostate cancer.

Tumor Stage

In order to be cured by radical prostatectomy alone, a prostate cancer must be confined within the margins of what can be excised surgically. The paucity of soft tissue surrounding the prostate does not allow wide surgical margins even in the best of circumstances. Therefore, tumors that breach the capsule of the prostate often are associated with positive margins. The following is a stage-by-stage discussion of the role of radical prostatectomy.

Stage T1a

T1a prostate cancers (by the Whitmore-Jewett classification) are low-volume tumors found incidentally at transurethral prostatectomy. In addition, a tumor must be low-grade in order to be included in this category. If the risk exposure is sufficiently prolonged, some stage T1a prostate cancers progress to clinical significance.[12,13] A repeat transurethral prostatectomy to gain additional staging information usually is not rewarding.[14] Sextant transrectal prostate biopsies may be helpful in detecting the minority of patients who harbor a significant residual volume of tumor within the prostate. Overall, however, radical prostatectomy is not indicated in patients with T1a tumors unless there is a likelihood of prolonged risk exposure.

Stage T1b

There is far less issue about the clinical relevance of T1b cancers compared to T1a lesions. Positive margins, if not positive pelvic nodes, are observed in over one-fourth of patients in most historical series.[15] However, the category of T1b is much less frequent now. Many of these patients are identified preoperatively by PSA testing. However, when T1b cancer is diagnosed, radical prostatectomy becomes appropriate treatment in patients with an expected survival of at least 10 years.

Stage T1c

Staging groups cancers into tumors with common characteristics and a presumed similar clinical prognosis. Most often, the common characteristics are size, depth of invasion, location, or extent of disease outside the site of origin. Stage T1c prostate cancer does not fit well into this scheme. The only characteristics common to stage T1c prostate cancers are histologically proven disease in a prostate gland considered benign by digital rectal palpation. A pertinent question, then, is whether categorizing cancers as T1c is a necessary convenience or a valid grouping of tumors which should be viewed and treated as a distinct entity.

Variability occurs within all clinical staging categories for prostate cancer or other tumors. There is no guarantee that palpable, T2b lesions are of the same size. In fact, it is well recognized that almost half of these are understaged clinically. However, variability within T1c tumors is more profound than with most other stages. A stage T1c cancer may be a small-volume, low-grade lesion in the transition zone or an extensive, high-grade tumor occupying the peripheral zone on both the right and left.[8]

Often, T1c cancers bear little resemblance to their closest neighbor on the staging algorithm, T1a or T1b.[5] By definition, at least a component of the latter is made up of transition zone tumor. Simultaneous tumor in the peripheral zone is, however, common even in T1a and T1b tumors. In fact, it has been suggested that it is the peripheral zone component which ultimately determines prognosis.

T1c cancer has been compared to T2a lesions with regard to treatment considerations. The volume and grade of the tumors in both categories (especially T1c) is variable but certainly overlaps.[16] The tumor is found pathologically to be confined within the prostate in the majority of men. There are, however, no real data to support or refute the notion that nonpalpable tumors have a prognosis and outcome similar to palpable lesions of a comparable size. The lack of alternative prognostic variables, though, prevents a clinician from making a distinction in projected outcome.[17] The similarity in treatment recommendations to men of comparable age and health who have histologically diagnosed palpable or nonpalpable cancers is more a matter of practical necessity and the consequence of an inability to identify valid distinguishing characteristics than any clinical information which shows equivalence between these cancers.

Stage T2

Palpable tumors apparently confined to the prostate historically have comprised the majority of most radical prostatectomy series. There are good data to show that T2 tumors progress both locally and with distant metastasis if observed for a sufficient period of time. On the other hand, when the surgical specimen shows a tumor confined within the prostatic capsule, surgical outcomes are excellent. Over 90% of patients with histologically confined tumors have undetectable PSA levels postoperatively and, apparently, are cured by radical prostatectomy.

The primary problem in selecting patients with T2 tumors for radical prostatectomy is identification of the significant percentage who are understaged clinically.[18] Almost 50% of T2b lesions are found to have extracapsular extension or positive margins. These patients are not cured by surgery alone. Unfortunately, though, no method has proven to be superior to digital rectal examination for staging the local extent of T2 cancers.

Endorectal magnetic resonance imaging provides excellent visualization of the prostate and, frequently, palpable tumors.[19] However, MRI scanning is expensive and not widely available. Furthermore, MRI staging of prostate cancer has not proven to be superior to transrectal ultrasound.[20]

In turn, transrectal ultrasound rarely provides any unique information compared to digital rectal examination.[6,21] Several features seen on TRUS are suggestive of tumor extension outside the prostate including marked asymmetry, interruption of the boundary echo, loss of some of the normal fat planes around the prostate, or a hypoechoic lesion in the seminal vesicle. However, it is unlikely that any imaging modality will be able to detect or predict with sufficient accuracy the microscopic amounts of tumor extension which often are present and limit the effects of treatment.[22]

Stage T3

Stage T3 tumors, by definition, have apparent local extension of tumor outside the prostate. As such, these patients are poor candidates for cure by radical prostatectomy. Although clinical overstaging may occur, especially after prostate biopsy, understaging is a far more common phenomenon. Radical prostatectomy has been performed for palliation of patients with known stage T3 cancers but there seems little justification for this on a routine basis.

Stage T1–2 N+

The finding of positive lymph nodes in patients explored for a planned radical prostatectomy is a far less common phenomenon than only a decade ago. This is a consequence primarily of earlier detection of prostate cancer and better patient selection, both driven primarily through the use of PSA. Nonetheless, positive pelvic lymph nodes may be encountered unexpectedly in patients felt to have tumors otherwise confined within the prostatic capsule. Radical prostatectomy alone is of no apparent benefit in this group of patients as they probably have subclinical distant metastasis. The role of radical prostatectomy with adjunctive therapy is discussed below.

PSA and Acid Phosphatase

Undoubtedly, serum markers now play a major role in selecting patients for radical prostatectomy. Often, it is an abnormality in PSA which leads initially to the diagnosis. In patients with known prostate cancer, numerous factors may influence the extent of PSA elevation, including tumor differentiation, volume, and, perhaps, vascularity and location.

Multiple other influences are probably operative but poorly defined. Despite this, there is a general correlation between the PSA level and the likelihood of extracapsular extension.[23] PSA levels in excess of 15–20 ng/ml are extremely worrisome for extracapsular extension regardless of the findings on digital rectal examination.[24]

What, then, should be the approach to a patient with a marked elevation in PSA? Patients with apparently localized disease but an elevated serum acid phosphatase have a generally poor outcome after radical prostatectomy even if the pelvic lymph nodes histologically are normal. Should a patient with a tumor apparently confined to the prostate on digital rectal examination but an abnormal acid phosphatase be excluded from radical prostatectomy?

There clearly is a subset of patients who have a very high PSA level and a large-volume tumor located primarily in the anterior portion of the gland which is still intracapsular. This, however, is rare. The substantial majority of patients with marked PSA elevations or any abnormality in acid phosphatase will ultimately be found to have extracapsular extension. Nonetheless, if the tumor is confined within the capsule by all other criteria, it becomes difficult to exclude these patients from radical prostatectomy if they are of young age and good health.

RADICAL PROSTATECTOMY AND ADJUNCTIVE THERAPY

If one accepts the premise that radical prostatectomy is curative only in patients with tumors completely excised by surgery, then there exists a disturbingly large group of patients who are not candidates for radical prostatectomy. Increasingly, though, for prostate cancer and other tumors, combination treatment is being used. Thus, it becomes pertinent to discuss the role of radical prostatectomy and adjunctive therapy.

Neoadjuvant Hormonal Therapy

Androgen deprivation decreases local prostate size in patients with carcinoma by 30–40%. This volume reduction is because of a decrease in size of both the benign and malignant portions of the prostate. Conceivably, then, neoadjuvant hormonal therapy could facilitate complete surgical excision of prostate cancer. It seems naive to expect neoadjuvant hormonal therapy to convert an extracapsular tumor to one entirely within the prostate. However, it is theoretically feasible that it would be easier to achieve negative margins by decreasing overall prostate size.

The data from several prospective studies on neoadjuvant therapy before radical prostatectomy are emerging.[25–27] Remarkably similar results have been found. The expected decrease in prostate size has occurred. However, there has been no evidence that the operation itself becomes technically easier. In fact, there may be increased difficulty with surgically removing the prostate gland after hormonal therapy. A substantial decrease in the histologic positive margin rate has been observed in several studies. A significant question, though, is how much of this is artifact. Histologic specimens become difficult to interpret after androgen ablation, especially at the margins of the tumor. There are not yet long-term survival or even PSA data demonstrating a superiority in outcome for patients undergoing neoadjuvant therapy.

In the absence of more definitive data, there does not seem to be sufficient justification for routine acceptance of neoadjuvant androgen ablation for radical prostatectomy. In particular, neither the available data nor logic support the use of neoadjuvant hormonal therapy and radical prostatectomy for patients with known T3 cancers. There may be a role in T2b lesions wherein a near 50% positive margin rate is observed without hormonal therapy, but further follow-up of ongoing studies is needed.

Adjuvant Hormonal Therapy

Although the use of neoadjuvant hormonal therapy is relatively new, adjuvant androgen deprivation has been used for many years, especially in patients with known residual disease or positive nodes.[28] As expected, there is a significantly prolonged time to disease progression or recurrence, but there still are no data to demonstrate an improvement in overall survival. Increasingly, though, there is a trend toward earlier clinical use of androgen ablation therapy based upon the belief that a longer response duration is observed if treatment is started when the disease is less bulky.

The role of the radical prostatectomy itself in this treatment algorithm must be questioned. If the premise of early hormonal therapy is accepted, does the surgery itself make a meaningful contribution to results? Tumor debulking is accomplished by surgery but death generally occurs because of distant disease. Nonetheless, the clinical significance of the cancer in patients with positive pelvic lymph nodes is not in question. This patient group has a poor long-term prognosis with delayed hormonal therapy alone. Efforts at early, aggressive treatment including hormonal therapy and surgical removal of the primary tumor seem justified in at least some patients until further data become available.[29]

Postoperative Irradiation

Radical prostatectomy removes the majority of cancer cells in patients found to have positive margins. Principles of radiation biology indicate that the best results with external beam irradiation are achieved in patients with small or microscopic volumes of disease. Using this logic, radical prostatectomy followed by postoperative irradiation becomes a reasonable planned treatment algorithm for patients found to have extracapsular extension.

There are, however, several limitations to this treatment approach. First of all, there is no evidence that surgical debulking followed by external irradiation is superior to radiation therapy alone. Furthermore, both treatments are limited by the recognition that many patients with extracapsular tumor extension fail because of distant disease despite apparent local control. In the absence of identifiable distant disease, though, postoperative irradiation seems appropriate for patients with known positive margins and/or detectable PSA after radical prostatectomy. However, a planned treatment algorithm of radical prostatectomy followed by external irradiation does not seem justified in the absence of data supporting this approach.

Salvage Radical Prostatectomy After Failure of Other Treatments

Patients undergoing external irradiation, interstitial brachytherapy, or cryotherapy may fail with intracapsular tumor recurrence or persistence. Theoretically, then, radical prostatectomy may still excise all remaining cancer. Several problems exist, though, in considering salvage radical prostatectomy.

First of all, it becomes even more difficult to determine whether the tumor truly is intracapsular. Often, after radiation therapy or cryosurgery, considerable fibrosis is present around the prostate, making an interpretation of digital rectal examination findings difficult. Also, a considerable number of these patients can be expected to have had local progression in the period of time between treatment and recognition of failure.

Undoubtedly, the morbidity and postoperative surgical complications for salvage radical prostatectomy are considerably higher than when the operation is performed in previously untreated men. Incontinence rates of over 25% are reported commonly and the risk of rectal injury is increased. Nerve-sparing approaches for retention of potency generally are not feasible.

Extreme caution should be used in selecting patients for salvage radical prostatectomy. Patients should not be subjected to the morbidity of the procedure unless there is a good likelihood that the tumor will be intracapsular and postoperative PSA levels undetectable. With careful patient selection, though, we have achieved undetectable PSA levels after salvage radical prostatectomy in the majority of our patients undergoing the procedure.

SURGICAL MORBIDITY AND EXPENSE

A requisite consideration in selecting patients for radical prostatectomy is the morbidity of surgery. Increasingly, patients become partners with the physician in the selection process. Although most men with a diagnosis of carcinoma of the prostate are deeply concerned about morbidity or death from the disease, they are also well aware of quality of life considerations. If treatment had no negative consequences, virtually all men would choose it regardless of whether it were proven to prolong life. The reality, of course, is that all treatments do have potential consequences which could impact negatively on quality of life.

The mortality rate from radical prostatectomy is less than 1% and major intraoperative complications are unusual. Blood transfusion is required rarely and the duration of hospitalization and cost of care have diminished substantially.[30,31] Potential loss of potency is a major treatment impediment for some patients but of no or little concern to many. Total incontinence is unusual but surgeons have failed to recognize or acknowledge previously the frequency or bothersome consequences of stress incontinence.

Clinicians are left with the problem of making treatment recommendations in the face of great uncertainty. Decisions should be made jointly with patients, individualized for each man, and unencumbered by external socioeconomic pressures. Radical prostatectomy is of proven benefit for some men with prostate cancer and the challenge remains in selecting men who are appropriate candidates for surgery.

REFERENCES

1. Sakr WA, Haas GP, Cassin FG, et al. The frequency of carcinoma and intraepithelial neoplasia of the prostate in young male patients. *J Urol* 150:379–385, 1993.

2. Stamey TA, Freiha FS, McNeal JE, et al: Localized prostate cancer: relationship of tumor volume to clinical significance for treatment of prostate cancer. *Cancer* 71:933–938, 1993.

3. Kabalin JN, McNeal JE, Price HM, et al: Unsuspected adenocarcinoma of the prostate in patients undergoing cystoprostatectomy for other causes: incidence, histology, and morphometric observations. *J Urol* 141:1091–1994, 1989.

4. Ohori M, Wheeler TM, Dunn JK, et al: The pathological features and prognosis of prostate cancer detectable with current diagnostic tests. *J Urol* 152:1714–1720, 1994.

5. Epstein JI, Walsh PC, Brendler CB: Radical prostatectomy for impalpable prostate cancer: the Johns Hopkins experience with tumors found on transurethral resection (stages T1a and T1b) and on needle biopsy (stage T1c). *J Urol* 152:1721–1729, 1994.

6. Hernandez AD, Smith JA Jr: Transrectal ultrasonography for the early detection and staging of prostate cancer. *Urol Clin North Am* 17:745–757, 1990.

7. Peller PA, Young DC, Marmaduke DP, et al: Sextant prostate biopsies: a histopathologic correlation with radical prostatectomy specimens. *Cancer* 75:530–538, 1995.

8. Scaletscky R, Koch MO, Eckstein CW, et al: Tumor volume and stage in carcinoma of the prostate detected by elevations in prostate specific antigen. *J Urol* 152:129–131, 1994.

9. Stamey TA: Making the most out of six systematic sextant biopsies. *Urology* 45(1):2–12, 1995.

10. Vallancien G, Prapotnich D, Veillon B, et al: Systematic prostatic biopsies in 100 men with no suspicion of cancer on digital rectal examination. *J Urol* 146:1308–1312, 1991.

11. McWhorter WP, Hernandez AD, Meikle AW, et al: A screening study of prostate cancer in high risk families. *J Urol* 148:826–828, 1992.

12. Epstein JI, Walsh PC, Eggleston JC: Prognosis of untreated stage A, prostate cancer: a study of 94 cases with extended followup. *J Urol* 135:242A, 1986.

13. Blute ML, Zincke H, Farrow GM: Long-term followup of young patients with stage A adenocarcinoma of the prostate. *J Urol* 136:840–843, 1986.

14. Parfitt HE Jr, Smith JA Jr, Gleidman JB, et al: Accuracy of staging in A, carcinoma of the prostate. *Cancer* 51:2346–2350, 1983.

15. Smith JA Jr, Gleidman JA, Middleton RG: Pelvic lymph node metastasis from prostate cancer: influence of tumor grade and stage in 452 consecutive patients. *J Urol* 130: 290–292, 1983.

16. Epstein JI, Walsh PC, Carmicheal M, et al: Pathologic and clinical findings to predict tumor extent of nonpalpable (stage T1c) prostate cancer. *JAMA* 271:368–374, 1994.

17. Irwin MB, Trapasso JG: Identification of insignificant prostate cancers: analysis of preoperative parameters. *Urology* 44:862–868, 1994.

18. McNeal JE, Price HM, Redwine EA, et al: Stage A versus stage B adenocarcinoma of the prostate: morphological comparison and biological significance. *J Urol* 139:61–65, 1988.

19. Quint LE, Van Erp JS, Bland PH, et al: Carcinoma of the prostate: MR images obtained with body coils do not accurately reflect tumor volume. *AJR* 156:511–516, 1991.

20. Ebert T, Schmitz-Drager BJ, Burrig KF, et al: Accuracy of imaging modalities in staging the local extent of prostate cancer. *Urol Clin North Am* 18:453–457, 1991.

21. Terris MK, Freiha FS, McNeal JE, et al: Efficacy of transrectal ultrasound for identification of clinically undetected prostate cancer. *J Urol* 146:78–84, 1991.

22. Flanigan RC, Catalona WJ, Richie JP, et al: Accuracy of digital rectal examination and transrectal ultrasonography in localizing prostate cancer. *J Urol* 152:1506–1509, 1994.

23. Lange PH, Ercole CJ, Lightner DJ, et al: The value of serum prostate specific antigen determinations before and after radical prostatectomy. *J Urol* 141:873, 1989.

24. Kleer E, Larson-Keller JJ, Zincke H, et al: Ability of preoperative serum prostate specific antigen value to predict pathologic stage and DNA ploidy. Influence of clinical stage and tumor grade. *Urology* 41:207, 1993.

25. Schulman CC, Sassine AM: Neoadjuvant hormonal deprivation before radical prostatectomy. *Clin Invest Med* 16(6):523–531, 1993.

26. Solomon MH, McHugh TA, Dorr RP, et al: Hormone ablation therapy as neoadjuvant treatment to radical prostatectomy. *Clin Invest Med* 16(6):532–538, 1993.

27. Labrie F, Dupont A, Cusan L, et al: Downstaging of localized prostate cancer by neoadjuvant therapy with flutamide and lupron: the first controlled and randomized trial. *Clin Invest Med* 16(6):499–509, 1993.

28. Zincke H, Bergstralk EJ, Larson-Keller J, et al: Stage D1 prostate cancer treated by radical prostatectomy and adjuvant hormonal treatment. *Cancer* Suppl 70:311, 1992.

29. Austenfeld MS, Davis BE: New concepts in the treatment of stage D1 adenocarcinoma of the prostate. *Urol Clin North Am* 17:867–884, 1990.

30. Koch MO, Smith JA, Hodge EM, et al: Prospective development of a cost-efficient program for radical retropubic prostatectomy. *Urology* 44(3):311–318, 1994.

31. Koch MO, Smith JA Jr: Impact of a collaborative care approach to radical retropubic prostatectomy. *Br J Urol* (accepted for publication).

2

Observation vs. Treatment for Localized Prostate Cancer

Bruce A. Lowe

Public awareness of prostate cancer has grown in recent years through educational efforts by a variety of national groups and greater media attention directed toward the disease. Coinciding with the advent of an enhanced diagnostic capability and the heavy penetrance in certain risk groups is an aging population resulting in the detection of substantially greater numbers of detected cases. The result has been a public perception of an epidemic that has affected nearly all either directly or through a relative or friend and threatens many more men.

Unfortunately, basic questions regarding the biologic behavior of this tumor and the capacity of available treatment modalities to affect natural progression and alter survival remain unanswered. As a result, the medical community is unable to reach a consensus regarding management. The public is confronted by a confusing barrage of mixed messages. Prestigious groups such as the American Cancer Society and the American Urological Association recommend annual screening evaluations for all adult males over 50 years of age, 40 years of age when a strong family history is present, while other equally prestigious groups such as the National Cancer Institute and the American Academy of Family Practice oppose this practice. Regardless of the validity of either position, the debate obscures the issues and each patient must choose amid conflicting opinions which course to pursue. When treatment success is uncertain, potential complications such as impaired voiding and sexual function may cause the patient to avoid any intervention. Recent attention has been directed toward several studies questioning the effectiveness of aggressive therapy and advocating watchful waiting. However, claims that prostate cancer is not a significant cause of morbidity and death are contradicted by the visible reality of frequent debilitation and tumor-related death common in the population and many individuals are willing to risk adverse results if cure is possible. Yet, the incomplete understanding of this disease leads to a vigorous debate and the voluminous available literature provides little in the way of verifiable answers. Treating physicians should be conversant in the pertinent issues in order to assist the patient in selecting the management course that is most likely to meet his individual needs and goals.

Primary care providers confronting these same issues face the same confusing dilemmas. A desire to offer a hope of effective treatment is offset by an increasing strain upon a system of limited resources. Failure to accurately define disease risk and treatment benefit heightens concern that therapy may not meet expectations and yet cause substantial morbidity. Faced with the responsibility of managing a vast array of medical needs, the generalist depends upon the specialist to provide concrete and verifiable answers to medical questions. When the experts are unable to agree, it is no wonder that primary care physicians and health care managers are unsure about the proper course. The large numbers of men at risk and subsequently found to have prostate cancer only compound the problem for these providers.

The following section reviews these issues. Though accurate and comprehensive answers are not possible, the discussion will review current understanding and outline an approach for selecting observation as the best option. Treatment goals should seek improved survival with an acceptable degree of morbidity or reduce the morbidity of untreated disease. Curative therapy attempts to accomplish these goals through eradication of the primary tumor. Observation or watchful waiting attempts to maintain quality of survival by avoiding needless treatment-related morbidity, especially when there is little or no evidence of treatment efficacy.

INCIDENCE OF PROSTATE CANCER

Before considering treatment selection, an understanding of the extent of disease in the population is necessary. With over 200,000 new cases detected during 1994, prostate cancer was not only the most common malignancy in men, but the most common noncutaneous malignancy in the United States. Even though the mortality rate is less than that seen with other leading cancers, the more than 38,000 deaths directly attributable to prostate cancer represent the second leading cause of cancer-related death in this country. In spite of recent advances in treatment and early diagnosis, the incidence and mortality rates have steadily risen for decades. However, the increase in incidence has been most marked in recent years with 165,000 new cases and 35,000 deaths reported during 1993 compared to 96,000 new cases and 27,000 deaths reported during 1987.[1] This represents a 108% increase from 1987 to 1994 for detection and a 40% rise in cancer-related deaths. Population growth of the United States during the same time was slightly over 5%. Most investigators believe this dramatic rise is due to enhanced diagnostic capability and the implementation of community-based screening programs.[2]

Simple improvements in the sensitivity of diagnostic procedures will increase detection because clinical prostate cancer represents only a fraction of the true incidence. Autopsy-based studies demonstrate histologic evidence of prostatic malignancy in over a third of 50-year-old men and in over one-half of 80-year old men studied.[3] Extrapolated to the general population, it can be presumed that subclinical disease exists in at least 10 million men in the United States alone.[4] However, only 2% of affected individuals are discovered during life and potentially at risk from their disease. Improved diagnosis will identify greater numbers of affected individuals, though it can be presumed that many will have subclinical disease of little potential impact. A newborn white male has a lifetime risk of developing clinical prostate cancer of 13.3% and 11.27% for an African-American male. Approximately 4% of men will die from this disease and nearly 3% of men alive today age 50 years and older will die from prostate cancer or a total of 900,000 men.[3] Risk is directly related to age and it can only be assumed that absolute incidence will continue to rise with the increasing median age of the national population. Carter and Coffey have estimated that the rise in detection will continue through the next decade and result in a 90% increase in incidence.[5]

SIGNIFICANCE

Approximately half of the men found to have prostate cancer will present with or subsequently develop disseminated disease with an expected 5-year survival of 32%.[6] A review of submitted Medicare claims demonstrated a 4.3-fold increase in the number of prostate biopsies and a 5.6-fold increase in the number of prostatectomies performed since 1987.[7] Yet even with improved detection resulting in aggressive treatment being provided to greater numbers of men, mortality rates continue to rise. Clearly, improved diagnostic capability has not resulted in improved survival. Increasingly it is apparent that prostate cancer is not restricted to the elderly. National surveys show that 18.4% of new cases occur in men less than 65 years of age, nearly 37,000 individual in 1994. It is not only the most common malignancy found in men in general, but in men less than 65 years of age and will cause the death of one-half of these younger individuals.[6]

The clinical course of prostate cancer is marked by slow local growth and eventual dissemination with gradual physical deterioration over a prolonged period. Local progression produces voiding dysfunction, pelvic pain, constipation, and urinary tract bleeding. These morbid conditions are concerning, but rarely threaten life. The slow wasting, cachexia, and escalating pain from bone metastasis have a greater impact upon the individual and require intensive management. Not only does disseminated disease adversely impact quality of life, but the side effects of treatment can be debilitating. The economic burden of diagnostic efforts and treatment of this common disease upon a health care system with limited resources is substantial, leading to increasing scrutiny by health care managers in both the private and government sectors.

THE EFFECT OF NATURAL HISTORY UPON TREATMENT SELECTION

Counseling a patient with prostate cancer requires the answer to two critically important questions. First, is treatment necessary? Second, if necessary to treat, then what therapeutic modality should be employed? In response to the first, if expected survival will be curtailed by uncontrolled growth of the cancer, then treatment is necessary. Treatment selected must be effective in eradicating disease while keeping morbidity to a minimum. To answer these questions requires an estimation of individual survival and a reasonable projection of tumor growth and progression. Such predictions are based upon assumptions that may be inaccurate. Recognizing that only 2% of all individuals with histologically evident disease will be detected during life and that less than 0.5% will experience a tumor-related death leads to the realization that not all patients require treatment to experience normal survival. Differentiating the significant from the insignificant lesion is problematic given current understanding of biologic behavior and the limits of technology. However, a number of very important studies provide the treating physician with reliable information upon which to base these predictions.

A basic tenet of oncology is that larger tumors are more likely to have local and distant extension at diagnosis and are associated with a poorer prognosis. The prognostic significance of tumor size is demonstrated by studies correlating capsular invasion and regional nodal involvement with tumor volume. Analysis of a series of prostatectomy specimens over a period of several years revealed that the majority of tumors less than 6-cc volume were not associated with either local or distant dissemination. Surgical excision would be expected to eradicate these cancers, whereas the great majority of tumors with volumes of 12 cc or greater are not curable.[8] These studies led to the presumption that prostate cancer arises as a small, relatively well-differentiated lesion that over time tends to increase in volume and becomes less differentiated. If correct, then early identification is the key to improving survival. These studies formed the intellectual foundation for the establishment of screening programs and as a consequence subsequent staging efforts focused on defining tumor volume, the smaller the lesion the greater the potential for cure.

Determining volume in the clinical setting is difficult and imaging studies, such as transrectal ultrasound and magnetic resonance imaging (MRI) have not led to improved staging accuracy, especially in the presence of microscopic extension. Transrectal sector biopsies were proposed as a method of mapping tumor volume and widely adopted. While this increases diagnostic yield, accuracy in defining tumor volume and predicting organ-confined disease is unproven. Attempts to correlate the number of biopsy cores demonstrating tumor with the frequency of extraprostatic disease found that the presence of malignant elements in more than one tissue sample was associated with local extension in 40%.[9] Other investigators noted the extent of core involvement roughly correlated with tumor volume. More than 2 or 3 mm of core involvement by tumor indicated a tumor volume greater than 0.5 cc.[10]

Recently questions over the validity of using tumor volume estimates to predict organ confinement have been raised by Epstein and associates who noted that many small-volume tumors exhibit higher grade disease.[11] Miller and Cygan analyzing 151 prostatectomy specimens with 293 tumor foci found many tumors with less than 1 cc total volume with Gleason scores of 8 to 10.[12] There was a strong correlation between tumor grade and microscopic stage. Nearly all Gleason score two lesions were organ-confined, 92% to 100%, regardless of volume, while high-grade tumors of Gleason score 8 through 10 were frequently extraprostatic, 86% to 96%. The nuclear differentiation criteria used by the National Prostatic Cancer Project (NPCP) grading system even more strongly correlated with disease extent with 97 of 106 (92%) grades 1 and 2 tumors being confined to the prostate, while 115 of 187 (61%) grades 3 and 4 tumors were extracapsular.[13] Another study found that well-differentiated tumors, grade 3 or less, were associated with nodal metastasis in less than 0.7% of patients, while lesions of grade 4 and 5 more than 4 cc in volume demonstrated nodal metastasis in 75% of patients. In one study grade and stage were shown to be interdependent parameters and could be used to predict future progression potential in individuals with clinically undetectable disease.[14] In a study of T1b tumors, final pathologic stage could not be accurately predicted unless the grade, volume, and location of the tumor were known.[15] From these studies, both grade and tumor volume are important parameters in predicting organ-confined and potentially curable disease and must be considered when selecting management.

Serum prostate specific antigen (PSA) levels are proportional to the volume of prostatic tissue and changes in these values can be correlated with changes in the volume of prostate tissue.[16] Stamey and associates followed PSA levels in 43 untreated patients and found steadily rising PSA levels in 86%, while only stable levels were seen in only 14%.[17] In the presence of organ-confined disease, PSA doubling time was greater than 24 months in 93%, 26 of 28 patients, and greater than 48 months in 60%. With extraprostatic disease the doubling time was greater than 24 months in only 53%, 8 of 15. Only 25% of patients with distant metastasis had PSA doubling times of greater than 24 months.[16] With this growth rate it would require more than 20 years for a single cell to develop into a 12-cc tumor. A 0.5-cc tumor attains a volume of 6 cc after approximately 10–12 years.[18] This validity of this growth model is supported by clinical studies. In 155 untreated T1 patients with microfocal disease, the median time to progression was 17 years. With extensive subclinical disease, the median time to progression was 4.7 years. Probability of progression was directly related to both grade and tumor volume.[14] Whitmore and associates followed 75 untreated patients with stages B1, B2, and B3 prostate cancer for mean intervals of 133, 130, and 108 months. Nearly all patients developed local progression within 60 to 70 months and this nearly always preceded the development of disseminated disease.[19] Malignant development may arise at a much earlier age than previously recognized as demonstrated by a recent autopsy study of young accident victims where the cellular changes characteristic of cancer were found in 27% of men ages 30 to 37 years and in 34% of men ages 40 to 47 years.[20] The presence of disease at such an early age throws into question the value of screening programs focusing on men over age 50 years.

EFFECTIVENESS OF TREATMENT IN ERADICATING DISEASE

Radical Prostatectomy

Effective treatment must be capable of completely eradicating disease. For many years clinical staging based upon digital rectal exams and later radionucleotide bone scans provided the objective information upon which staging was determined and treatment selection based. While recognizing that many undergoing prostatectomy or radiotherapy would suffer treatment failure, most patients were considered cured and expected to remain disease-free. When careful pathologic examinations of prostatectomy specimens became standard, it was discovered that many clinically localized tumors were actually extraprostatic and not eradicated by surgical resection. Extraprostatic disease manifested by capsular perforation or involvement of the surgical margin was reported in 18% to 48% of prostatectomy specimens.[15,21] A review of 571 patients undergoing radical prostatectomy for clinically localized disease found organ-confined disease in only 61% of the surgical specimens. Regional nodal involvement was noted in 65, or 11%, and extraprostatic extension or T3 disease in 161, or 28%.

Improvements in imaging devices and techniques held the promise of improved staging accuracy, however a number of investigators have been unable to consistently identify pathologic stage using transrectal ultrasound or MRI studies. Neither has been found to improve staging over PSA and digital rectal exams. In addition, most periprostatic tumor extension in the absence of palpable extension by digital rectal exam is microscopic and difficult to identify by any available imaging technique.

The proven ability of PSA to improve detection of prostate cancer and monitor treatment effectiveness has prompted investigations into using the test in tumor staging. Oesterling and associates found PSA to be a strong predictor of metastasis with levels less than 20 ng per ml only rarely associated with disease-related lesions demonstrated by bone scan.[22] Routine use of bone scans in the presence of PSA levels less than 20 ng per ml will seldom identify dissemination.[23] A bone scan in newly detected prostate cancer should be done only in those patients at risk if indicated by other clinical findings. Additional support for the use of PSA was provided by Catalona and associates when they found levels tended to be greater than 10 ng per ml in the presence of extraprostatic disease and less than 10 ng per ml in most patients with organ-confined tumors.[24]

Treatment-related morbidity following prostatectomy occurs in only a minority of patients. Yet, for many men the potential loss of urinary control and sexual function is unacceptable and many decline treatment because of this risk or to seek alternatives. Recent advances in surgical technique, a greater understanding of pelvic anatomy, and improved surgical skill through a combination of training and increased experience have substantially decreased perioperative complications. Most institutions report mortality rates of less than 0.5% following radical prostatectomy and one large series including over 3,000 procedures did not experience a single perioperative death.[25] Another review of 1,324 men undergoing pelvic lymphadenectomy and total prostatectomy reported three perioperative deaths for a mortality rate of 0.2%.[26] In 571 prostatectomies performed by 11 different surgeons in four separate facilities over a 6-year period, there were three operative mortalities for a 0.5% mortality rate. These studies demonstrate that surgical excision of the prostate is attended by a low risk of perioperative mortality in both community and academic centers.

Quality of life following prostatectomy for most individuals is dependent upon the successful recovery of urinary continence and sexual function. Stress urinary incontinence following prostatectomy is reported by nearly all major centers to occur in less than 10% of patients. Total urinary incontinence is uncommon. Complete urinary control following prostatectomy is reported in 92% of patients and mild incontinence requiring the wearing of one pad per day or less noted in 6%.[27] Improved surgical exposure gained via an anatomic prostatectomy as described by Walsh[28] can significantly reduce postprostatectomy incontinence. In one study postprostatectomy incontinence was 6% in patients undergoing an anatomic prostatectomy compared to 30% in those undergoing a nonanatomic procedure.[27] In some centers postprostatectomy incontinence is reported to be 5%.[29]

Sexual activity in men is dependent upon the intact function of two separate nerve pathways. Erectile function is dependent upon the integrity of the cavernosal pathway described by Walsh and Donker.[30] Injury to these nerves during prostatectomy will result in erectile failure. Many men are functional at diagnosis and desire to remain sexually active. Preservation of the cavernosal nerves at the time of prostatectomy can maintain erectile function in many men. In a recent update of the Hopkins series, 68% of all men with adequate function before surgical excision were potent 18 months after a nerve-sparing procedure. For men less than 50 years of age, 91% maintained erectile function, while 75% of men 50 to 60 years of age and 58% of men 60 to 70 years of age were able to do so. Preservation of erectile function beyond age 70 years was less than satisfactory with only 25% maintaining potency.[29] In properly selected patients nerve-sparing prostatectomy is not associated with an increase in detectable tumor at the surgical margin.

Morbidity from surgical excision of the prostate is low and usually manageable. Andriole and associates reported 98 nonfatal early complications following 1,324 prostatectomies (7.2%) requiring treatment. Thromboembolic events were the most common and seen in 34 or 2.6%, cardiovascular events in 19 or 1.4%, wound problems in 17 or 1.3%, and miscellaneous complications in the remainder.[26] Bladder neck contractures are reported in 4% to 10% of patients. A trend toward increased frequency of operative morbidity was seen with advancing age, but this did not achieve statistical significance.

Radiation Therapy

Since the introduction of the linear accelerator in the early 1960s, external beam radiotherapy has played a major role in the management of prostate cancer. Attempts to reduce treatment-related morbidity and deliver larger radiation doses targeted specifically to the prostate prompted development of interstitial implantation of radioisotopes into the prostate. Reports that the complications and success of treatment were less than hoped for, coinciding with the advances in surgical technique, resulted in a movement away from radiation therapy toward radical prostatectomy.[6,18,32] However, technological and procedural advances in the delivery of radiation have renewed interest in this treatment modality in managing these tumors.

The Stanford group recently reported on the long-term results of radiotherapy in 1,245 patients with clinically localized prostate cancer. In 690 individuals with clinical stage T1 and T2a and unknown nodal status, survival was 40% at 15 years and cause-specific survival was 68%.[33] In a review by Hanks and associates of the Pattern of Care Studies (PCS) and Radiation Therapy Oncology Group (RTOG) trials, the 15-year actuarial survival of patients with stage T1 prostate cancer after external beam radiotherapy was no different than expected survival of an age-matched population. In stage T2 disease, survival was approximately half of expected.[34] Most radiotherapy studies are hampered by incomplete staging with accurate tumor status unknown at the time of treatment. Consequently, many centers restrict treatment to patients with a high probability of organ-confined disease by not offering therapy when pretreatment PSA levels are greater than 20 or 40 ng per ml, considered an indication of eventual treatment failure.[35]

Cytotoxic effects of ionizing radiation develop over an ill-defined time period and not all prostatic tissue is destroyed. Normalization of the digital rectal exam once used to monitor treatment success is an inadequate parameter for measuring outcome. Needle biopsy of the prostate following radiation demonstrates residual disease in 12% to 91% of individuals.[36] However, biopsies performed to monitor the tumor status may be misleading if obtained too soon after treatment. Residual carcinoma detected by needle biopsy 2 years or longer after therapy correlates with a high degree of recurrence and is a strong indication of treatment failure.[18,37] One prospective study of 143 patients found residual tumor in 19% of T1 patients and 28% of T2b patients 2 years after completion of treatment.[35] Postirradiation PSA levels are subject to errors in interpretation because of the presence of residual nonmalignant prostate tissue, however, increasing PSA levels following radiation is an adverse prognostic sign and indicative of active tumor growth.[38] Failure of PSA levels to normalize by one year after treatment is a sign of active residual disease and is associated with a high incidence of recurrence.[22,39] Paralleling the results seen with radical prostatectomy series, postirradiation PSA levels will be detectable in many individuals with clinical resolution of disease. In 269 patients with clinical organ-confined cancer treated by external beam radiotherapy, PSA levels decreased in virtually all patients initially for 9 months. However, failure of the serum PSA to drop below 1.0 nanogram per milliliter at the nadir was nearly always accompanied by eventual treatment failure and was seen in nearly 52% of patients.[35]

Morbidity of radiotherapy is low and using conventional techniques a treatment mortality of 0.2% can be expected. Severe complications will occur in 1.9% and usually involve the urinary and gastrointestinal tracts. Erectile dysfunction occurs in 45 to 61% of patients. Subsequent urinary incontinence will develop in 0.9%. Bladder neck contracture or urethral strictures are found in 4.1% and are often associated with a history of prior transurethral resection of the prostate. Acute irritation to the gastrointestinal tract manifested by diarrhea, tenesmus, and rectal bleeding is noted in approximately 36% of patients.[17] Recent efforts to reduce morbidity and improve tolerance through the use of conformal techniques demonstrate patients' tolerance of higher doses with reduced toxicity. One study using conformal therapy reported only two severe complications in 324 patients, 0.6%, and minor complications in 15% and 34% respectively.[40]

Alternative Therapy

The controversy surrounding treatment efficacy stimulates increased efforts to identify alternative therapies that may offer improved survival or maintain current survival rates with lower morbidity. Investigational therapies include transurethral laser ablation, hyperthermia, and cryosurgery. Interstitial radiation, or brachytherapy, utilizes new technology in an effort to improve delivery and reduce complications. Though these methods offer attractive theoretical benefits, it is not appropriate to recommend one as a first choice without ensuring the patient understands the investigational nature of these modalities. Interstitial radiation was found to be less than satisfactory 10 years ago and recommending its use in other than investigational protocols is unethical.[41] Cryosurgery trials are being initiated in many centers and preliminary studies indicate this modality may have a definite role for small-volume tumors, as adjuvant treatment for persistent disease following radiotherapy, or in patients who are not candidates for other modalities.[42]

OBSERVATION IN THE MANAGEMENT OF LOCALIZED PROSTATE CANCER

Expectant management has been commonly employed for the management of prostate cancer in selected patients for many years. Advocating an expanded role for observation is not a new concept. However, observation is used frequently in this country and is illustrated by the American College of Surgeons surveys during the 1980s reporting that 65.7% of patients with stage A (T1) disease were managed expectantly and that 16.7% of patients with stage B (T2) disease received no curative treatment. Another 6% with stage A and 9% of stage B tumors were managed by androgen deprivation alone. When taken together, in 1985, 32.2% of all patients in the United States with clinically localized disease were managed by observation.[6] The current controversy centers on patient selection and treatment effectiveness. Conventional wisdom advocates withholding treatment from the individual with limited survival or from the older patient where prolonged survival is unlikely. However, many treating physicians are not following these historic precedents. Recent reviews of Medicare data show marked increases in billing codes for diagnosis and treatment submitted for patients over 75 years of age. Active treatment in this group may be inappropriate and a poor allocation of resources.

A number of published studies report the international experience with observation in managing patients with prostate cancer. Widely cited by the media and many public health leaders as evidence for restricting the application of aggressive management to only a few select individuals, many of the criteria used in these studies are of concern. Selection criteria for entry are not uniform, but nearly all of these studies include significant numbers of individuals with small-volume and well-differentiated tumors. Patients entering observation trials are selected from larger groups. Results of these treated patients are usually not provided in the reports. No prospective randomized study comparing observation and treatment arms has yet been published. The same inaccuracies and potential selection bias that plague treatment studies exist with observation trials. The only valid conclusion that can be drawn from these studies is that not all patients with clinical disease will require treatment in order to avoid cancer-related mortality. As noted previously, this is not a new revelation. However, these studies are valuable in clarifying the need for more complete information regarding natural history and treatment efficacy. Finally, the mean age of the subjects in nearly every study is high and usually over 70 years of age. Many patients included in these studies would not be considered candidates for treatment in the United States and this further weakens the power of the conclusions. Therefore, universal extension of observation to all individuals with prostate cancer may be inappropriate. A brief summary of the major observation studies reported is given below.

Handley and associates managed 278 asymptomatic patients by observation, 20% of these having disseminated disease at enrollment. During a mean follow-up of 41 months 49% experienced local progression requiring interventional therapy. Cancer-related deaths were very high in this study, occurring in 45% of those patients developing progression, and are due to the inclusion of a large number of patients with metastasis.[43] In another prospective study of 120 patients with clinically localized disease reported by George, mean age was 74.8 years and the duration of follow-up was less than 5 years. Although 82% of patients developed local progression, only 23 patients or 19% required treatment to relieve outlet obstruction and 11% progressed to metastatic disease. A total of 44% died during the study, but only 4% died from prostate cancer. This difference in cause-specific death is not surprising given the advanced age of many patients in the group and underscores the importance of this parameter in determining survival.[44]

Adolfsson and associates reported a retrospective review of 122 untreated patients with well or moderately well-differentiated clinically localized disease, 13 stage T1 and 109 stage T2. Median age was 68 years. The median length of follow-up was 81 months. During follow-up 55 patients (45%) required treatment for progressive tumor, with androgen deprivation utilized in 36, external beam radiation in 12, radical prostatectomy in 4, and interstitial I-125 in 3. Risk of local progression at 5 years was 57% and 8% developed metastases, while at 10 years local progression occurred in 69% and metastasis in 28%. Cancer-related death occurred in 16% of patients at 10 years and another 31% died from unrelated causes. A recent update of the series included an additional 50 patients and extended the mean follow-up to 99 months. Local progression was seen in 58%, but only 22% required treatment to relieve obstruction. Disease-specific survival at 10 years was 80%.[45]

The study by Johansson and associates has generated the greatest amount of discussion. A total of 223 of 654 new cases of prostate cancer, mean age 72 years, were followed without treatment. The majority of tumors were grade 1 and 106 of 223 or 48% were stage T0, 72 stage T01, and 34 T0d. In a recent update of the results, progression was seen in 77 patients (35%), and 28 (13%) developed metastasis. Androgen deprivation therapy was instituted in 64 patients, or 28%. A total of 148 patients died (66%) but only 23 (10%) died from prostate cancer.[46]

Whitmore and associates reporting on 75 patients with clinical stage B disease found that local progression would eventually develop in all patients, if followed for a sufficient period of time. In 29 patients with B1 disease the mean time to local progression was 63 months, 78 months for the 37 patients with stage B2 disease, and 175 months for nine stage B3 patients. During a mean follow-up interval of 133 months, 13 of 29 or 45% of B1 patients required treatment specifically for management of local progression. Seven or 24% received treatment directed at the primary tumor and six developed distant disease. Six patients died, two from myocardial infarction, one with metastasis, and four from prostate cancer at a mean of 150 months. During a mean follow-up of 130 months, 26 of 46 (56%) stage B2 and B3 patients required treatment for local progression and 23 died, five from cardiovascular disease while receiving endocrine therapy and nine due to cancer.[19]

Moskovitz and associates followed 101 untreated patients, mean age 72 years, with a mean follow-up period of 58 months. All patients underwent either open prostatectomy or transurethral resection. Five-year survivals for stages T0b, T1–2, and T3 were 91%, 61%, and 42% respectively.[32] Kolon and Albertsen identified 698 patients not undergoing therapy with curative intent from the Connecticut Tumor Registry between the ages of 65 and 85 years of age. In this group survival was not dependent upon age. In patients given androgen deprivation therapy alone, a cancer-specific mortality of 20% to 27% was seen at 10 years. Cause-specific 15-year survival by Gleason grade was G2–4: 82–93%, G5–7: 67–78%, G8–10: 46–57%.[47]

INDIVIDUAL PATIENT SURVIVAL PROJECTIONS

When recommending management options, individual survival potential in the absence of prostate cancer must be considered. Average life expectancy for a white male in the United States during 1992 was over 73 years and under 70 years for an African-American male. Obviously, not all men die in their mid 70s. However, a healthy 70-year-old male can expect an average of 9 to 11 additional years. In addition, longevity is increasing as annual death rates for American men continue to decrease by 1.5% per year. Currently 5% of the population is over 80 years of age and this is steadily increasing. Consequently, it may not be appropriate to withhold aggressive therapy from a healthy man in his early or mid 70s. Physicians must consider each individual's potential life expectancy when recommending treatment. Life tables compiled by the insurance industry indicate that a 60-year-old man in good health can expect a 5-year survival rate of approximately 90%

and a 15-year survival of approximately 70%.[48] Death due to cardiovascular causes has been steadily decreasing in the United States since 1964, whereas the mortality rate due to cancer, including prostate, and infection, primarily HIV is increasing. By the year 2000, 13% of the population will be over age 65 years. Death from prostate cancer will be an increasingly important health consideration in the next century. When estimating patient survival, comorbidity of intercurrent illness must also be considered. Expected survival is reduced by 50% if the patient suffers from poorly controlled angina or has had a recent myocardial infarction. Insulin-dependent diabetes, poorly controlled hypertension, and a low performance status will be associated with an increase in mortality of approximately 30%.[49,50]

SELECTING THE PATIENT WITH LOCALIZED DISEASE FOR OBSERVATION

From the preceding discussion it is apparent that treatment selection should depend upon predictions of tumor growth and progression compared to estimated survival. When potential disease progression will adversely affect survival, aggressive intervention should be considered. It is often stated that treatment should only be offered to individuals with a survival potential of greater than 10 years. However, this generalization may not be applicable to the individual with a high-grade, low-volume tumor that will progress without treatment in less than 5 years and yet is organ-confined. Curative therapy may offer improved survival with better quality of life for these individuals than could be achieved through expectant management. However, the low mortality and morbidity rates currently reported with treatment are due to patient selection and should be restricted to those patients able to tolerate these procedures with minimal risk. Poor performance status or significant comorbidities would be contraindications to aggressive therapy. In these patients, the cost of treatment related morbidity versus the potential survival advantage is unjustified.

For the overwhelming majority of patients undergoing curative treatment for prostate cancer, impact upon quality of life is of greatest importance and urinary incontinence is more concerning than erectile impotence. However, expectant management does not guarantee that quality of life will be unaffected. Given sufficient time, nearly all tumors will progress locally and many will require operative intervention to relieve obstruction or control bleeding. Androgen deprivation therapy will be instituted in many patients and is not without complications. The attendant side effects can often be quite severe and debilitating. These adverse events are more likely to occur in the younger individual due to the longer intervals for tumor growth. In these patients, observation is really delayed therapy and the morbidity of local and distant progression may impact quality of life to the same degree as aggressive intervention. However, the differential impact of treatment on quality on life versus observation has not been adequately studied.

Selecting Patients with T0 Disease for Observation

Low-grade microfocal disease, stage T01, is associated with a prolonged interval between diagnosis and progression, usually more than 10 years. Active treatment for healthy patients over 75 years of age or younger individuals with moderate comorbidity is not necessary to maintain survival. When a similar lesion is present in a younger man, a treatment plan that meets management goals is less obvious and the crux of the issue is not whether to intervene, but when. Immediate intervention may impact quality of life long before the cancer threatens survival. However, delaying therapy without compromising survival depends upon the accuracy of initial staging and subsequent monitoring of tumor growth. Any error may lead to disease progression before treatment can be instituted and possibly increase morbidity and tumor-related death. In this situation, staging must employ both meticulously performed imaging studies and multiple sector biopsies to confirm the presence of small-volume disease. If more extensive disease is not discovered after these efforts, observation may be an appropriate option. The individual desiring this course must be aware that current diagnostic tools are imprecise and that errors in clinical staging may occur, leading to an increased potential for treatment failure.

The optimal timing of PSA levels and transrectal ultrasound studies with guided biopsies required to follow those individuals choosing observation is not yet known. In addition, it is unknown whether multiple biopsies over time will increase the risk of extracapsular disease through tract seeding or increase postprostatectomy morbidity due to traumatic fibrosis. Further study is required to define these possible risks. A less definable adverse consequence of observation described by individuals choosing this option is the psychological impact of living with an untreated growing cancer. Many patients initially choosing this option will subsequently request treatment because of the anxiety induced by the waiting.

Grade 8 to 10 lesions will usually progress in less than 5 years and will require more aggressive treatment to prevent tumor-related death. Younger healthy patients with high-grade T01 or T0d, regardless of grade, should be advised to seek curative therapy. Those choosing observation should be followed carefully and often, with immediate intervention whenever tumor growth or grade migration is detected. The older patient over 70 years of age with limited survival potential or significant intercurrent illness will only require supportive measures.

Selection of Patients with T1–2 Disease for Observation

The substantial numbers of clinically localized tumors exhibiting extraprostatic disease at excision and the frequency of PSA-detected failure, even in the presence of pathologically proven organ-confined disease, leads many to believe that active intervention will not benefit the majority of patients with prostate cancer. Further, the slow growth of these tumors may negate the value of treatment in those with truly organ-confined disease. However, many of these patient will experience progression without treatment and need tumor eradication to achieve a lasting disease-free survival. The primary difficulty is not in the capability of therapy to accomplish this, but in selecting individuals who need and will benefit from treatment. Obviously more sensitive diagnostic and staging modalities are needed.

As noted previously, individual survival potential is the crucial factor in selecting patients for observation. Individuals with limited survival need no additional treatment and can be watched expectantly. Again, tumors that are small and well-differentiated will be associated with prolonged intervals before undergoing progression. Observation may be an option for these patients as in those with T01 disease. Conversely, healthy individuals with high-grade disease and good survival potential should be offered treatment. However, a 25% to 35% incidence of extraorgan disease will be found in these patients. Though survival is compromised by this finding, prolonged survival before dissemination will occur in the majority of these patients. In a review of the author's experience, less than 20% of patients with stage T3a–b lesions will experience local progression or disseminated disease in 5 years.

Treatment recommendations should be made after careful consideration of individual survival potential and projected tumor growth. Unnecessary intervention will be minimized when offered only to those with a possible survival greater than expected without the adverse effect of the cancer. Restricting therapy to this low-risk population will be most likely associated with improved survival and the lowest degree of morbidity. In addition, providing observation to the younger patients willing to accept a slightly higher risk of disease progression will select out for subsequent treatment those individuals with a greater potential for extended survival.

REFERENCES

1. Seidman H, Mushinski MH, Gelb SK, et al: Probabilities of eventually developing or dying of cancer. *CA* 35:36–56, 1985.
2. Corder EH, Chute CG, Guess HA, et al: Prostate cancer in Rochester, Minnesota (USA), from 1935 to 1989: increases in incidence related to more complete ascertainment. *Cancer Causes and Control* 5:207–214, 1994.
3. Sakr WA, Haas GP, Cassin BF, et al: The frequency of carcinoma and intraepithelial neoplasia of the prostate in young male patients. *J Urol* 150:379–385, 1993.
4. Lubke WL, Optenberg SA, Thompson IM: Analysis of the first-year cost of a prostate cancer screening and treatment program in the United States. *JNCI* 86:1790–1792, 1994.
5. Carter HB, Coffey DS: The prostate: an increasing medical problem. *Prostate* 16:39–48, 1990.
6. Mettlin CJ, Murphy G: The National Cancer Data Base report on prostate cancer. *Cancer* 74:1640–1648, 1994.
7. O'Donnell PD, Finan BF: Continence following nerve-sparing radical prostatectomy. *J Urol* 142:1227–1229, 1989.
8. Shipley WU, Zietman AL, Hanks GE, et al: Treatment related sequelae following external beam radiation for prostate cancer: a review with an update in patients with stages T1 and T2 tumor. *J Urol* 152:1799–1805, 1994.
9. Ackerman DA, Barry JM, Wicklund RA, et al: Analysis of risk factors associated with prostate cancer extension to the surgical margin and pelvic node metastasis at radical prostatectomy. *J Urol* 150:1856–1850, 1993.
10. Dietrick D, McNeal J: Needle core cancer length and cancer volume estimation in small cancers of the prostate. *J Urol* 292A, 1994.
11. Epstein JI, Carmichael MJ, Partin AW, et al: Small high grade adenocarcinoma of the prostate in radical prostatectomy specimens performed for nonpalpable disease: pathogenetic and clinical implications. *J Urol* 151:1587–1592, 1994.
12. Miller GJ, Cygan JM: Morphology of prostate cancer: effects of multifocality on histological grade, tumor, volume and capsule penetration. *J Urol* 152:1709–1713, 1994.

13. Miller EB, Ladaga LE, el-Mahdi AM, et al: Reevaluation of prostate biopsy after definitive radiation therapy. *Urology* 41:311–316, 1993.

14. Lowe BA, Listrom MB: Incidental carcinoma of the prostate: an analysis of the predictors of progression. *J Urol* 140:1340–1344, 1988.

15. Epstein JI, Walsh PC, Brendler CB: Radical prostatectomy for impalpable prostate cancer: the Johns Hopkins experience with tumors found on transurethral resection (stages Ta1 and T1b) and on needle biopsy (stage T1c). *J Urol* 152:1721–1729, 1994.

16. Stamey TA, Freiha FS, McNeal JE, et al: Localized prostate cancer: relationship of tumor volume to clinical significance for treatment of prostate cancer. *Cancer* (Suppl) 71:933–938, 1993.

17. Schmid H-P, McNeal JE, Stamey TA: Observations on the doubling time of prostate cancer. The use of serial prostate specific antigen in patients with untreated disease as a measure of increasing cancer volume. *Cancer* 71:2031–2040, 1993.

18. Scardino PT, Wheeler TM: Local control of prostate cancer with radiotherapy: frequency and prognostic significance of positive results of postirradiation prostate biopsy. *Natl Cancer Inst Monogr* 7:95–103, 1988.

19. Whitmore WF Jr, Warner JA, Thompson IM Jr: Expectant management of localized prostatic cancer. *Cancer* 67:1091–1096, 1991.

20. Olsson CA, Goluboff ET: Detection and treatment of prostate cancer: perspective of the urologist. *J Urol* 152(part 2):1695–1699, 1994.

21. Kabalin JN, McNeal JE, Johnstone IM, et al: Serum PSA and the biologic progression of prostate cancer. *Monographs Urol* 16(1):1–16, 1995.

22. Oesterling JE, Martin SK, Bergstraih EJ, et al: The use of prostate-specific antigen in staging patients with newly diagnosed prostate cancer. *JAMA* 269:57–60, 1993.

23. Walsh PC, Donker PJ: Impotence following radical prostatectomy: insight into etiology and prevention. *J Urol* 128:492–497, 1982.

24. Catalona WJ, Smith DS, Ratliff TL, et al: Detection of organ-confined prostate cancer is increased through prostate specific antigen-based screening. *JAMA* 270:948–954, 1993.

25. Zincke H, Oesterling JE, Blute ML, et al: Long-term (15 years) results after radical prostatectomy for clinically localized (stage T2c or lower) prostate cancer. *J Urol* 152:1850–1857, 1994.

26. Andriole GL, Smith DS, Ganeesh R, et al: Early complications of contemporary anatomical radical retropubic prostatectomy. *J Urol* 152:1858–1860, 1994.

27. Steiner MS, Morton RA, Walsh PC: Impact of anatomical radical prostatectomy on urinary continence. *J Urol* 145:512–515, 1991.

28. Walsh PC: Radical retropubic prostatectomy. In Walsh PC, Gittes RF, Perlmutter AD, et al (eds): *Campbell's Urology*, ed 5. Philadelphia, WB Saunders, 1986, vol 3, pp. 2754–2775.

29. Igel TC, Barrett DM, Segura JW, et al: Perioperative and postoperative complications from bilateral pelvic lymphadenectomy and radical retropubic prostatectomy. *J Urol* 137:1189–1191, 1987.

30. Walsh PC, Donker PJ: Impotence following radical prostatectomy: insight into etiology and prevention. *J Urol* 128:492–497, 1982.

31. Walsh PC, Partin AW, Epstein JI: Cancer control and quality of life following anatomical radical retropubic prostatectomy: results at 10 years. *J Urol* 152:1831–1836, 1994.

32. Moskovitz B, Nitecki S, Richter-Levin D: Cancer of the prostate: is there a need for aggressive treatment? *Urol Int* 42:49–52, 1987.

33. Bagshaw MA, Cox RS, Hancock SL: Control of prostate cancer with radiotherapy: long-term results. *J Urol* 152:1781–1785, 1994.

34. Hanks FE, Hanlon A, Schultheiss R, et al: Early prostate cancer: the national results of radiation treatment from the patterns of care and radiation therapy oncology group studies with prospects for improvement with conformal radiation and adjuvant androgen deprivation. *J Urol* 152:1775–1780, 1994.

35. Zagars GK: Prostate specific antigen as an outcome variable for T1 and T2 prostate cancer treated by radiation therapy. *J Urol* 152:1786–1791, 1994.

36. Zietman AL, Shipley WU, Coen JJ: Radical prostatectomy and radical radiation therapy for clinical stages T1 to T2 adenocarcinoma of the prostate: new insights into outcome from repeat biopsy and prostate specific antigen followup. *J Urol* 152:1806–1812, 1994.

37. Scardino PT: Problem of prostate cancer. *J Urol* 152:1677–1678, 1994.

38. Russell KJ, Dunatov C, Hafermann MD, et al: Prostate specific antigen in the management of patients with localized adenocarcinoma of the prostate treated with primary radiation therapy. *J Urol* 146:1046–1052, 1991.

39. Kaplan ID, Cox RS, Bagshaw MA: Prostate specific antigen after external beam radiotherapy for prostatic cancer: followup. *J Urol* 149:519–522, 1993.

40. Leibel SA, Zelefsky MJ, Kutcher GJ, et al: Three-dimensional conformal radiation therapy in localized carcinoma of the prostate: interim report of phase 1 dose escalation study. *J Urol* 152:1792–1798, 1994.

41. Nag S, Scaperoth DD, Badalament R, et al: Transperineal palladium 103 prostate brachytherapy: analysis of morbidity and seed migration. *Urology* 45:87–92, 1995.

42. Miller RJ Jr, Cohen JK, Merlotti LA: Percutaneous transperineal cryosurgical ablation of the prostate for the primary treatment of clinical stage C adenocarcinoma of the prostate. *Urology* 44:170–174, 1994.

43. Handley R, Carr TW, Travis D, et al: Deferred treatment of prostate cancer. *Br J Urol* 62:249–253, 1988.

44. George NJ: Natural history of localized prostatic cancer managed by conservative therapy alone. *Lancet* i:494–497, 1988.

45. Adolfsson J, Bonstrom L, Lowhagen T, et al: Deferred treatment of clinically localized low grade prostate cancer: the experience from a prospective series at the Karolinska Hospital. *J Urol* 152:1757–1760, 1994.

46. Johansson J-E: Expectant management of early stage prostate cancer: Swedish experience. *J Urol* 152:1753–1756, 1994.

47. Kolon TF, Albertsen PC: Conservative treatment of clinically localized prostate cancer: fifteen year survival analysis stratified by age and histologic grade at presentation. *J Urol* 149:229A, 1993.

48. 1983 Group Annuity Mortality Table. *Trans Soc Actuaries* 35:859–900, 1992.

49. Schellhammer PF: Contemporary expectant therapy series: a viewpoint. *Urology* 44:47–52, 1994.

50. Woolf SH: Public health perspective: the health policy implications of screening for prostate cancer. *J Urol* 152:1685–1688, 1994.

3

External Beam Radiation Therapy in the Treatment of Prostate Cancer

Martha K. Tibbs
Anthony L. Zietman
William U. Shipley

External beam radiation therapy has often been employed as the definitive treatment in a large proportion of men who present with clinical stage T1 and T2 adenocarcinoma of the prostate. In a number of institutions it also represents the primary treatment for patients who present with more locally advanced T3–4 tumors.[1]

In evaluating the efficacy of radiation as a definitive treatment, the definition of a treatment failure must first be established. Failure following external beam irradiation was, until the late 1980s, defined as the development of palpable disease at the primary site or of clinically evident distant metastases. Recently, more rigorous and more controversial endpoints have been debated. These have developed, firstly, from the routine use of serum prostate specific antigen (PSA) in follow-up and, secondly, from the policy of some institutions to rebiopsy prostates at intervals after irradiation.

SERUM PSA

The early detection of failure following treatment for any cancer has potential uses. Because biochemical failure often precedes clinical failure by months to years, post-therapy PSA levels may assist in the evaluation of new treatment strategies over 5 years rather than over decades. PSA levels may also help to limit the confounding effect of competing morbidity in this often elderly population. In addition, and on an individual basis, salvage therapy may be instituted early with this sort of information available. Most physicians now agree that a sharply rising PSA constitutes failure, however, disagreement persists as to what represents a normal level following radiation therapy and in what time interval such a level should be achieved.

Following radical surgery, the PSA level is expected to remain undetectable if disease is controlled. Following radiation therapy, the PSA had not been expected to fall below

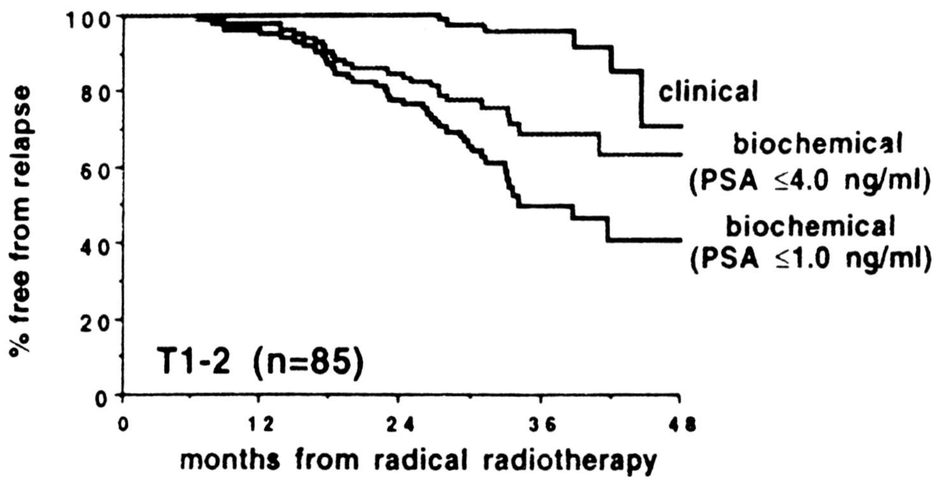

Fig. 3.1. Freedom from clinical and biochemical relapse for T1 and T2 patients. Chemical failure is shown using both the top of the normal PSA range and the more stringent criteria that is increasingly judged more appropriate.

detectable levels as the argument has been made that residual prostate tissue persists and remains capable of producing PSA. Initially, it was felt that if the level was between 0 and 4 ng/ml, which represents the normal limits of the general population, treatment had been effective. However, high-dose radiation therapy is known to diminish protein synthesis in other glands, so it is likely that it would demonstrate the same effect in prostatic tissues. Indeed, a recent report by Willett et al.[2] found that even when a normal prostate received incidental radiation in the course of treating another pelvic malignancy, its ability to produce PSA was diminished. A more reasonable estimate of a normal level following radiation is actually less than 1.5 ng/ml, and perhaps less than 1.0 ng/ml.

PSA follow-up has significantly reduced the estimation of cure for any local therapy and appears to result in a 25% lower disease-free survival than reported previously based on clinical grounds (Fig. 3.1). The use of hormonal therapy has an independent effect on the PSA level, and the interpretation of serum PSA following the increasingly common combinations of radiation and neoadjuvant androgen suppression is yet to be clarified.

POSTRADIATION REBIOPSY

Kuban studied 94 patients who had a negative digital rectal exam after radiation therapy and who underwent rebiopsy at least 18 months later.[3] Those with T1b disease had a 10% rate of positive rebiopsy, those with T2 18%, and those with T3–4 21%. By 10 years the clinical local failure rate was 75% for those patients with positive biopsies and the disease-free survival 20%. Those who had a negative postradiation biopsy had a local failure rate of only 30% and a disease-free survival of 60% over the same interval. In considering these results, it is crucial to realize that no attempt was made to judge the viability of the tumor cells present in the positive biopsy specimens. A positive biopsy specimen with a declining or normal PSA may not have biologically active disease, and any residual tumor deposits may still be responding to treatment.[4] Cellular death following exposure to radiation is a postmitotic event. As many prostate tumors have a long doubling time, cells that have been lethally damaged may not yet have had the opportunity to express this damage morphologically. Biopsies may therefore be interpreted as positive for many months or even years.

The likelihood of a positive postradiation biopsy is correlated with initial Gleason grade, initial stage, PSA (Fig. 3.2), techniques of irradiation, total dose, method of postradiation biopsy, and the presence or absence of abnormality on digital rectal examination.[5,6] At the Massachusetts General Hospital, 37 men who had received irradiation for T3 prostate tumors underwent a postirradiation biopsy.[6] These were men without local failure, who had 24 months or more follow-up, and who had received no endocrine therapy. Overall, 62% had a negative biopsy and 38% had a positive biopsy. Of moderate to well-differentiated tumors, 79% had a negative biopsy, and of poorly differentiated tumors, 36% had a negative biopsy. Of patients with PSA less than 2.5 (19 patients), 79% had a negative biopsy, and of patients with a PSA greater than 2.5 ng/ml (14 patients), 29% had a negative biopsy. There was a low probability of a positive postradiation biopsy in men with a normal prostate by digital rectal exam and a normal serum PSA.

The correlation of postradiation biopsy results with survival has been inconsistent and even its true incidence uncertain. Its implications therefore remain controversial.[1,6]

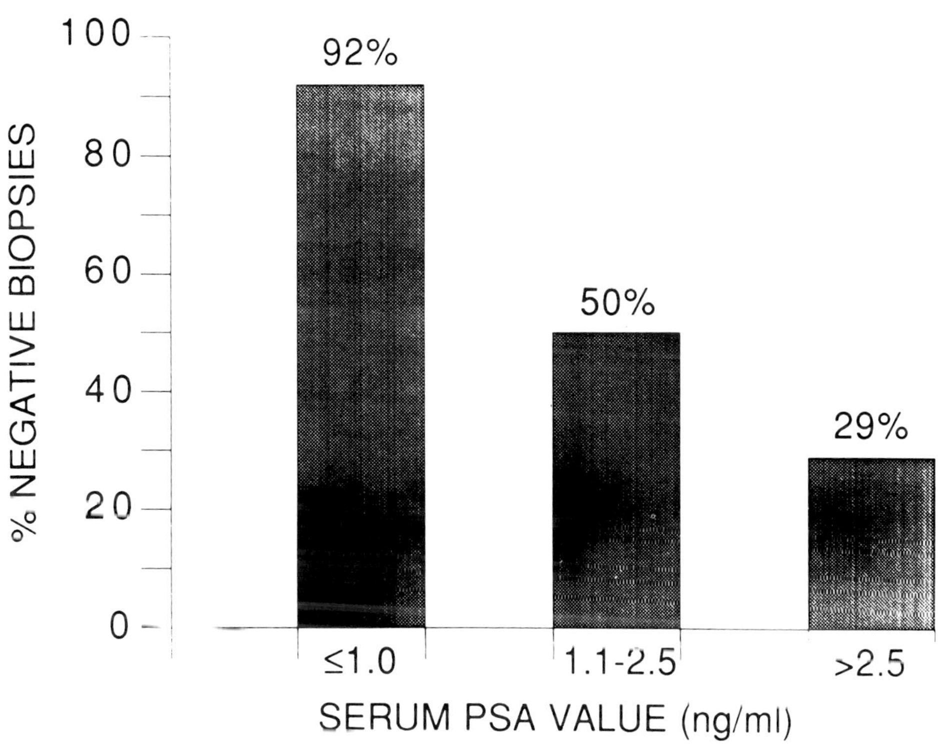

Fig. 3.2. Proportion of men with negative postradiation biopsies as a function of the PSA at the time of rebiopsy in a group of 33 men.

EARLY STAGE DISEASE: T1 AND T2 TUMORS

"Early stage disease" has generally included those tumors felt to be organ-confined and corresponds to the clinical T1 and T2 classification. It is a term loosely used to encompass a heterogeneous and diverse subgroup of patients with regard to biologic aggressiveness and curability by radical monotherapy. It is considered by some a category in substantial need of redefinition. Often it includes patients with high initial PSA levels (>10–15 ng/ml), high Gleason grades (sums of 8–10), and stages T2b–c tumors none of which are well served by any single currently available therapy.

In radical prostatectomy series, the surgeons have the advantage of choosing young patients in good medical condition and of obtaining a staging lymphadenectomy prior to performing prostatectomy. In radiation series, the patients tend to be older with less than ideal medical conditions, and frequently they have more extensive local tumors even within the T1–2 category. In radiation therapy series, the lymph node status is most often unknown. For an optimal comparison of the results of surgery and radiation, all patients would ideally be surgically staged or be randomized before receiving treatment based on the findings of their various staging procedures. As this is rarely possible, careful consideration of the proportions of patients with unfavorable characteristics must be made prior to any comparisons between series.

At the Massachusetts General Hospital (MGH), the patients with clinical stages T1 to T2 disease treated between 1988 and 1991 were retrospectively analyzed.[5] Of those receiving radiation, 54% were found to be T2b–c and fully one-third had a PSA greater than 15. Of those receiving surgery, 41% were T2b–c but only 11% had a PSA greater than 15. Patients with higher grade tumors and higher PSAs were more likely to receive external beam radiation therapy. The proportion of such patients within any series can influence outcome as profoundly as the local therapy itself. In the MGH series, men with an initial PSA of less than 15 ng/ml had a 64% chance of remaining biochemically disease-free at 4 years compared with less than 10% for those with values greater than 15 ng/ml (Fig. 3.3).

A number of large series have recently reported lengthy follow-up for conventional external beam irradiation. These provide the measure against which improved radiation strategies, including the implant and conformal therapy, can be judged.

The Radiation Therapy Oncology Group (RTOG) undertook a prospective randomized study to evaluate elective nodal radiation in T1b to T2 patients whose lymph node status was determined by lymph node dissection.[7] Of 104 patients with node negative disease who would have qualified as surgical candidates, the survival exceeded the aged matched expected survival for 10 years of observation (63% as compared with the expected 59%). The outcome was equal to long-term reports of the radical prostatectomy in similarly staged patients. In the RTOG series, 87% of patients were free of isolated local recurrence, 79% were free of metastatic failure, 67% were free of any failure, and 86% were free of cancer deaths at 10 years. The local control rate at 10 years was 84%, and 79% were without distant metastases at 10 years. Of the long-term clinical disease-free survivors, 85% had a serum PSA below 1.5 ng/ml, and 65% below 1 ng/ml.

In the Patterns of Care study, T1N0 tumors showed no excess mortality after 15 years following radiation, a condition which satisfies a strict definition of cure.[7,8] For T2 tumors there was an excess mortality continuing to 15 years after radiation which was 20 per-

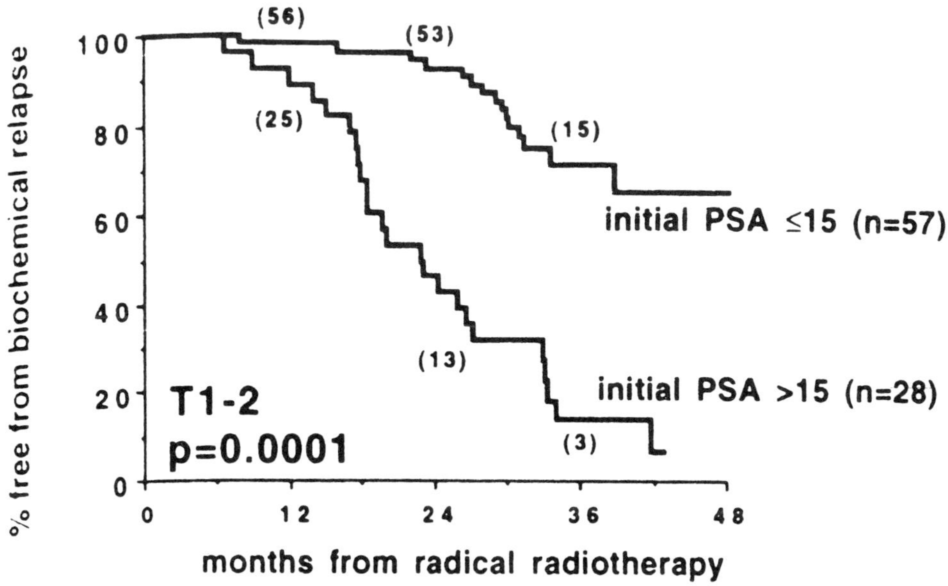

Fig. 3.3. Likelihood of freedom from biochemical failure at 4 years for T1 and T2 patients based on pretreatment PSA. Those with an initial PSA below 15 ng/ml fared significantly better.

centage points below expected. For stage T2 patients, 22% were alive at 15 years with two-thirds clinically free from disease. Small-volume cancers were considered cured with radiation except for a small subset with positive lymph nodes. Intermediate volume cancers required observations beyond 15 years, to find a return to expected mortality. This pattern is suggestive of a slow progression with an unusually long and natural history and implies that radiation may postpone mortality by effecting temporary cytoreduction. Large-volume cancers represent disease that is not controlled and may follow a more progressive course with an excess mortality at 5 years which is gone by 10 to 12 years.

Lee and Sause reported on 71 patients with T1b–2 N0 disease and noted 92% actuarial local control at 15 years.[9] Also at 15 years 40% were clinically disease-free, and none had a PSA above 1.4 ng/ml.

Schellhammer et al. showed 40% clinical disease-free survival at 10 years but when serum PSA was taken into account this fell to less than 20%.[10] Better results were obtained for those with T1–2a tumors and tumors of lower grade.

Zietman et al. studied over 500 men treated over the 1980s and also reported biochemical disease-free survival below 40% for the T1–2 group overall.[11] When the T1–2a well–moderately differentiated subgroup ("surgical candidates") are analyzed separately, the 10-year figure exceeded 50% (Fig. 3.4).

In Bagshaw's experience from Stanford with 1,245 men who were treated with external beam radiation for prostate cancer between 1956 and 1992, the staging system was consistently applied and the Gleason grading was adopted early, making this series unparalleled in the literature.[12] In this mature analysis, the overall median survival was 10 years. With such complete follow-up over more than two decades, PSA determinations were unnecessary. The best results were obtained in T1 and T2a patients with negative

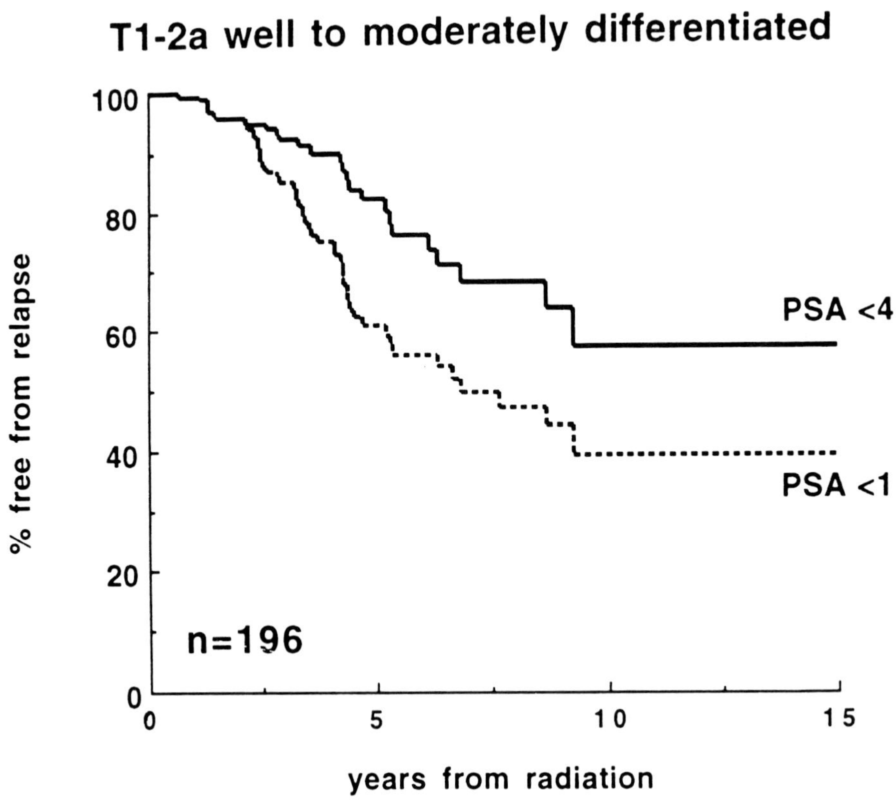

Fig. 3.4. Actuarial freedom from biochemical relapse in a subgroup of patients from MGH radiation series who are comparable to those considered surgical candidates.

lymph nodes who achieved a 53% 15-year survival, which was identical to an age matched cohort of men without prostate cancer. The cause-specific survival at 15 years for all stages of tumors was 52%. For T1a and T1b tumors there was no statistically significant difference in survival as compared with an age matched control population. For T2a tumors the survival pattern was also identical with 50% survival at 15 years. T2b and T2c tumors fared worse than T2a. Survival after relapse was 40% at 5 years, 18% at 10 years, and 9% at 15 years, and was longer for those patients who relapsed in their prostate or who had well-differentiated tumors.[12,13]

A recent controversial publication by Stamey described a series of 98 patients who received external beam radiation therapy.[14] He found that only 43% of T1 patients and 20% of T2 patients were free from a rapidly rising PSA with 5 years of follow-up. His study has been widely criticized, as within the T2 category he made no distinction between those with T2a, T2b, or T2c disease nor did he report the initial Gleason grades or pretreatment PSA values. It is likely that these were very high and that, for this group of patients, radical prostatectomy would have produced similarly poor results.[11]

Using controls matched for age, stage, and Gleason grade, Freiha, like others from Stanford including Stamey and Bagshaw, has compared radiation with retropubic radical prostatectomy.[15] It was found that at 10 years, survival for radiation patients was 75%

with 8 of 53 dead of disease at a minimum of 10 years. Survival for radical prostatectomy patients was 85% with 4 of 53 dead of disease between 7 and 11 years. In this comparison, statistical significance between the two modalities was not reached. Dr. Stamey's apocalyptic vision of 80% or more of patients failing clinically by 10 years does not seem to have been borne out either by the Freiha or the Bagshaw reports despite their lengthy follow-up.

In conclusion, long-term results therefore show a high probability of cure for men with true early disease (T1–2a, Gleason ≤ 6, PSA < 15 ng/ml) using conventional external beam irradiation. Men with poor prognostic features, however, usually fail when conventional dose external beam is used alone.

LOCALLY ADVANCED DISEASE

Twelve to 28% of newly diagnosed prostate cancers are stage T3–4. Urologists tend to refer these locally advanced prostate cancer patients for radiation in order to avoid taxing surgery when the possibility of cure is slim. While the primary goal of radiation therapy in these men is cure, more realistic goals are the prolongation of survival and the prevention of local progression with a minimum of morbidity.

Using conventional external beam radiation, cure rates are usually below 20% at 10 years.[16] They are lower still for those with high initial PSA values and Gleason grades. The clinical local recurrence rate for these bulky tumors at 10 years has been estimated at between 20% and 60%.[13,17,18]

Stanford reported a 10-year survival of 35% in T3 patients and an 18% 15-year survival rate.[12] M.D. Anderson reported a 45% 10-year survival and a 31% 15-year survival in similar patients.[13] Washington University reported a 42% 10-year survival in T3 patients.[18] Clearly room exists for improvement in therapy.

Recent attempts to improve this outcome have focused on increasing the accuracy of the treatment delivered, safely increasing the radiation dose delivered, and adding short- or long-term androgen suppression.[1,19,20] Better local control and more effective systemic agents will both be necessary before any great improvements in survival are seen.

The most appropriate radiation field and the benefits of highly targeted "conformal" therapy remain unsettled. Differences of opinion have surrounded the use of elective irradiation of the pelvic lymph nodes. It is expected that 40% to 50% of T3–4 tumors would be accompanied by positive pelvic lymph nodes if lymphadenectomy were performed.[7] Some institutions have chosen to minimize the size of their standard fields and eliminate pelvic lymph nodes from the volume of tissue treated, their justification being that if the disease has progressed to the lymph nodes it is more than likely present at distant sites as well. The majority of studies, however, show improved pelvic control for patients with T3–4 tumors when the pelvic lymph nodes are included in the radiation field, but none show improved survival.[1,18]

These studies have also demonstrated the importance of treatment accuracy as tight inferior field margins were associated with significantly lower pelvic control rates.[18] Corn et al. have shown that accurate targeting of radiation improves biochemical disease-free outcome for T1–3 patients at 3 years when compared with historical controls treated conventionally.[21] This advantage came without any increase in dose delivered, and hopefully will translate into a durable therapeutic gain.

The higher the delivered radiation dose, the higher the probability of local tumor control. This holds for most human tumors, and prostate cancer is not an exception. Hanks reporting for the Patterns of Care Study showed that doses greater than 65 Gy have yielded better results for T3–4 patients.[7] Patients who received less than 60 Gy had a 37% 5-year clinical local recurrence rate. It was 36% for those patients receiving 60 to 64.9 Gy, and 29% for those receiving 65 to 69.9 Gy. Those who received more than 70 Gy had a 5-year local recurrence rate of 19%.

The only randomized trial so far that has looked at dose escalation was reported in 1995 by Shipley et al. from the MGH. A phase 3 high-dose versus conventional dose external beam radiation therapy trial was undertaken for stages T3 and T4 disease. A 12.5% increase in dose using a proton boost to 75.6 cobalt Gy equivalents (CGE) by a conformal perineal approach was used. Proton therapy is based on the deposition of energy or dose by a beam of monoenergetic protons which increases slowly with depth but reaches a sharp maximum peak near the end of the particle's range, called the Bragg peak period.[20] This trial was conducted between 1982 and 1992 with 103 patients receiving 75.6 cobalt Gy equivalent and 99 patients receiving 67.2 Gy using conventional techniques. Overall there was no change in survival, recurrence-free survival, or local control (Fig. 3.5). The latter did show a trend toward an advantage for the higher dose. A subgroup, however, the poorly differentiated patients, showed significantly increased local control with high dose, 85% as compared with 37% at 7 years (Fig. 3.6). The proton boost improved local control but also increased late sequelae. A higher incidence of grade 1–2 rectal bleeding

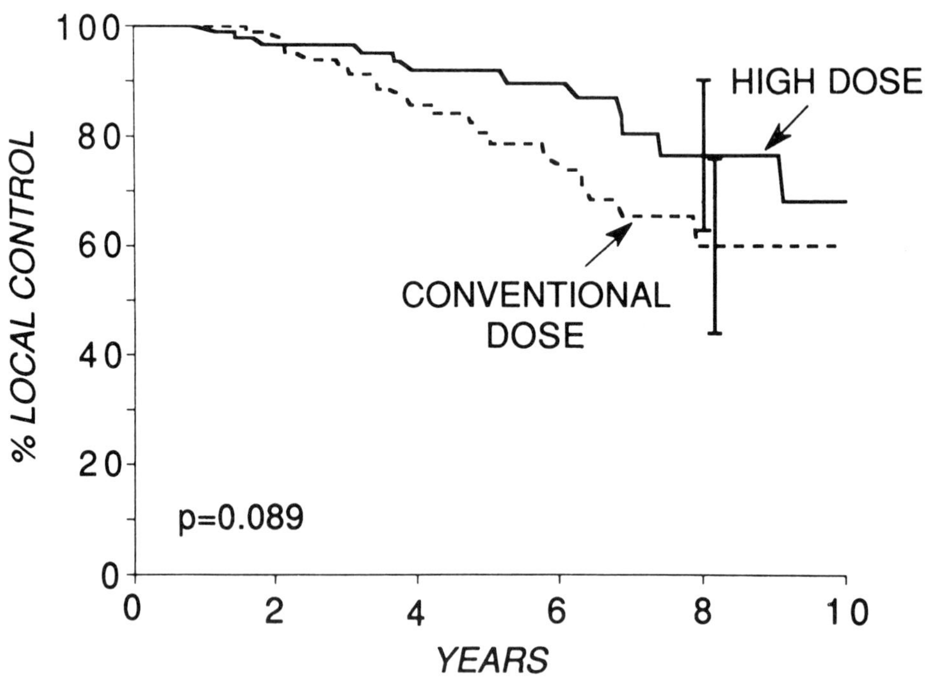

Fig. 3.5. Kaplan-Meier estimate of local control in patients receiving high-dose irradiation with a conformal proton boost as compared with those receiving a conventional dose with photons alone (n = 189).

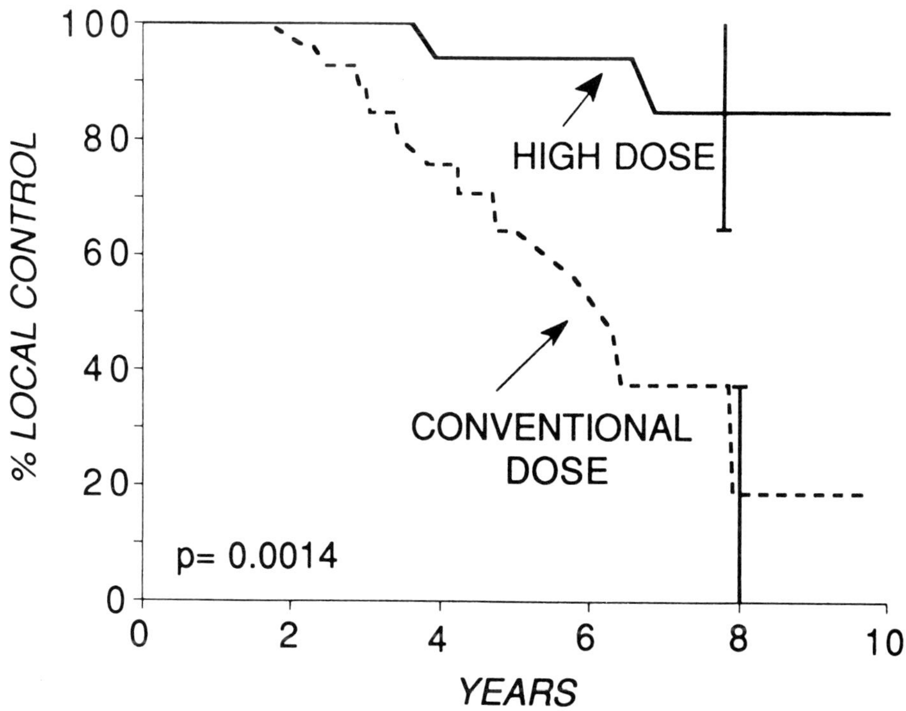

Fig. 3.6. Kaplan-Meier estimate of local control for patients with poorly differentiated tumors who received either high-dose irradiation incorporating a conformal proton boost or conventional photon irradiation (n = 57).

was noted in the high-dose arm.[22] This may be a small price to pay if a genuine survival advantage could be proven.

Androgen suppression as an adjunct to radiation has been utilized firstly, in an attempt to deal with occult metastatic disease (adjuvant therapy), and secondly, for cytoreduction in patients with bulky tumors prior to radiation in order to enhance the probability of local tumor control (neoadjuvant therapy). Androgen suppression reduces tumor volume and probably clonogen number resulting, it is speculated, in increased tumor control for a given radiation dose.

In the randomized trial RTOG 86-10, an attempt to reduce tumor volume prior to radiation was made using neoadjuvant androgen suppression.[23] This study examined 455 patients with T2b–4 disease. In the experimental arm, total androgen blockade was given for 2 months prior to and during irradiation and compared with the same irradiation scheme alone in the control arm. The local recurrence rate was significantly lower in patients treated with neoadjuvant androgen suppression at 5 years compared with the control group (Fig. 3.7) as was freedom from all failure including PSA failure. There was only a trend toward an advantage in terms of distant metastases, but this may become more evident with the passage of time. There was no difference in overall survival nor morbidity between the two arms. The benefit of 4 months of neoadjuvant androgen suppression was evident many years after the discontinuation of therapy, supporting the hypothesis that combined modality results in improved tumor cell killing.

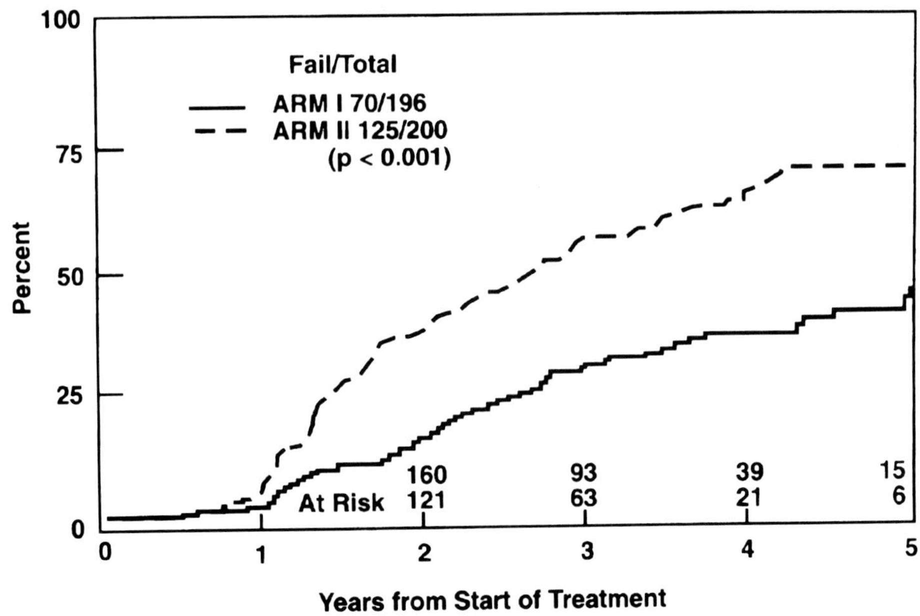

Fig. 3.7. Incidence of local progression by treatment arm in RTOG 86-10. Arm I consisted of pre-treatment androgen blockade combined with radiation. Arm II patients received the same radiation therapy without hormonal treatment.

RTOG study 85-31 compared adjuvant goserelin following radiation with radiation alone in clinically staged T3 patients.[24] At 5 years the actuarial incidence of local failure was 17% for the adjuvant androgen suppression group and 32% for the observation group. The 5-year actuarial rate of distant metastasis was 19% for the experimental group and 29% for the observation group. At 5 years, the percentage of men with no evidence of disease and with a PSA less than 1.5 ng/ml was 49% for the experimental group and 17% for the observation group. All of these differences are statistically significant. The 5-year actuarial survival rate was 76% for the experimental group and 71% for the observation only group, a value that did not reach statistical significance.[24,25]

The RTOG has initiated a new trial, 9202, in which all patients receive neoadjuvant androgen suppression but half also receive 2 years of maintenance suppression after radiation therapy is complete. The endpoint will be freedom from biochemical failure.[1]

POSTOPERATIVE IRRADIATION

The benefits of prostatectomy are mainly limited to those patients with organ-confined disease. Detecting these patients in advance may be difficult due to the limitations of clinical staging. Up to 26% of patients who have clinical T1b disease may be upstaged to pathologic T3 at the time of radical surgery.[26] For those with T2a tumors, upstaging may be found in 33%. Only around 40% of clinically staged T2b–c patients are found to have organ-confined disease at the time of surgery.

Pathologic T3 tumors may be subcategorized according to their extent. These categories correlate with prognosis and patterns of failure and include: capsular penetration; seminal vesicle involvement; and positive surgical margins. Surgical margins are more likely to be positive if tumors extend outside the capsule but may also occur if the capsule is incised during a difficult dissection, which is particularly likely to happen at the prostatic apex and occurs in up to 23%.[26] Of men with extracapsular disease, a positive surgical margin, or seminal vesicle involvement 45% to 75% will relapse within 5 years after radical prostatectomy.[27–29]

Data from Duke University draw a clear distinction between specimen-confined pT3 disease and positive surgical margins with 4-year recurrence rates of 32% and 66% respectively.[28] The investigators at Johns Hopkins have distinguished between focal and extensively positive surgical margins. Those with only focally positive margins show a 40% progression at 5 years whereas those with extensive positivity of surgical margins show a 65% progression at 5 years.[30] Detectable PSA following surgery may be an indicator of persistent local disease, in which case radiation is currently the treatment of choice. Alternatively, it may be an indicator of metastatic disease, in which case androgen suppression would be more appropriate.

Adjuvant irradiation is commonly recommended for those men with positive surgical margins and for those with extensive extracapsular disease who have negative lymph nodes and no seminal vesicle involvement. These men are at high risk for failure and there is a high probability that it will be local. If the seminal vesicles are involved, the expectation of success is lower following radiation, as seminal vesicle involvement frequently correlates with the presence of distant metastases.[30] If lymph nodes are involved, most failures are metastatic disease.[27] Radiation may reduce local failure but offers little chance of cure in this latter group of patients.

If the probability of local failure is high, it intuitively seems most appropriate to irradiate the tumor bed at the time that the residual tumor is smallest in volume, i.e., adjuvant treatment. Link has suggested that deferring radiation until the PSA level has begun to rise may result in less potential for cure and may be too late for these men.[31] Morbidity from tumor regrowth at the site of prostatectomy includes bladder outlet obstruction, pain, hematuria, and ureteral obstruction. Allowing regrowth also permits a second possibility for the development of distant metastases. In addition higher doses of radiation are required for larger tumor burdens.[27] Adjuvant radiation has been advocated postoperatively for those with involved surgical margins even with an undetectable PSA. These men are likely to benefit from treatment and demonstrate 50% to 70% freedom from biochemical failure at 5 years.

In a study from the University of Southern California, 71% of men who underwent radical retropubic prostatectomy had a positive surgical margin or showed evidence of seminal vesicle involvement. For these men, the 4-year freedom from biochemical relapse following postoperative irradiation was 66%.[32] Freeman has reported on 114 patients in whom the disease-specific survival and overall survival improved as compared with historical controls when radiation was added to those patients found to be pathologic T3 following retropubic prostatectomy.[32] In a series from Meier who made a nonrandomized comparison, men who received adjuvant irradiation had a local failure rate at 10 years of 6% and a metastatic rate of 9%.[33] Those who did not receive irradiation had a 10-year local failure rate of 31% and a metastatic rate of 45%. McCarthy, in his series from Washington University, analyzed 64 men who received postoperative irradiation for pT3 disease, a detectable PSA, or both. Of these, 67% of the men were without relapse at a median follow-up of 27.5 months.[34]

Early adjuvant radiation has also been advocated at Massachusetts General Hospital.[35] Postoperative radiation was delivered to 68 men with pathologic T3 disease, 50 of whom had positive surgical margins. The freedom from biochemical failure at 5 years was 64% for those with positive surgical margins and 43% for those with seminal vesicle involvement.

The principal concern about postoperative adjuvant irradiation is that some patients are undoubtedly treated unnecessarily having either no residual surgical bed disease or occult metastases. In addition, it has not been clearly demonstrated to improve survival. This may in part be due to the extended natural history of the disease with competing morbidities of men in this age group which would obscure any benefit.[30]

Now, with the use of PSA, we have the opportunity to observe pT3 patients and can attempt salvage irradiation at an early stage when the PSA starts to rise. Salvage irradiation has a good chance for success in those who had involved margins at the time of their surgery. Lower success is found in those who had involved seminal vesicles, poorly differentiated tumors, and a PSA above 2 to 3.[30] Salvage irradiation reduces PSA levels in 80% of men, and 50% have a reduction in their PSA to undetectable.[36] Unfortunately only one-quarter to one-third remain free from biochemical failure at 5 years.[27,31,32,34,37,38]

MORBIDITY OF EXTERNAL BEAM THERAPY

There is a low incidence of serious complications associated with external beam irradiation (Table 3.1). Sequelae may be divided into the acute and the chronic. Acute are those occurring during treatment. They are common but the majority are self-limiting. Chronic sequelae persist after the completion of radiation and represent reactions of vascular connective tissue and parenchymal tissues to injury. Mild or moderate symptoms are those that are transient and modest enough to be well controlled with simple medications. Severe symptoms require surgical intervention, prolonged hospitalization, or are life-threatening.[39]

Typical acute sequelae that occur during conventional irradiation include fatigue, urinary frequency, dysuria, and rarely urinary retention. Diarrhea, mild proctalgia, and occa-

TABLE 3.1. Summary of Complications Following Radiation Treatment for Prostate Cancer

Adverse Event	*Incidence after Radical Radiation*
Lethal complication	< 1 per 1,000
Severe complication	< 1%
Severe rectal injury	< 1%
Severe incontinence	0.4–4%
Stricture	1–11%
Loss of potency	32–67%

sional rectal bleeding are also noted. One or more of these side effects occur in one-third to one-half of patients undergoing irradiation treatment for prostate cancer.[39]

Patients are, however, more often concerned about potential chronic sequelae. Most chronic symptoms with the exception of incontinence and impotence are not persistent but occur only for a number of weeks or months before they subside or are corrected by minor surgical procedures.[39] A number represent subacute inflammatory reactions. Urinary incontinence occurs overall in less than 1% of men who were continent prior to radiation at 5 years of follow-up. It is more common among those who underwent TURP.[39,40] Incontinence is often preceded by one or more TURPs in an attempt to correct symptomatic bladder neck contraction or stricture at the urethra. After high-dose irradiation if a TURP is performed, healing may be poor and therefore compromise the integrity of the external sphincter.[39] For patients who receive postoperative radiation after prostatectomy, the recovery of continence was not affected beyond any difficulties attributed to surgery.[11,30,32,39,40]

The issue of potency is also a concern for patients. Thirty to 60% retain full potency following prostate irradiation.[1,39] Erectile dysfunction after radiation has been attributed to induced endarteritis of branches of the internal pudendal and penile vessels which course lateral to the prostate and are in the high-dose region.[41] Other potential urologic side effects that occur in a small percentage of men include hemorrhagic cystitis, bladder contracture, or urethral stricture.[39,42,43]

Rectal bleeding occurs to some degree in approximately 10% and is a direct function of the volume of the anterior rectal wall within the radiation field and the dose it receives.[39,44] Symptoms generally resolve with stool softeners and steroids. Anal strictures and chronic diarrhea were observed in less than 1%.[18,42]

Infrequent sequelae include genital or leg edema which occurs in less than 1% of patients and is an extremely rare complication with radiation alone. After surgery, 10–30% of patients may experience this complication if they are treated with whole pelvic irradiation following a lymph node dissection.[1]

CONVENTIONAL AND MODERN RADIATION TECHNIQUES

Several retrospective studies have indicated the importance of radiation dose and its effect on local control. Typically tumor doses have ranged from 60 to 64 Gy for T1a tumors, 65–70 Gy for T1b and T2 tumors, and 70–72 Gy for T3.[1] It is important to consider the appropriate dose and volume based on the patient's stage of disease, pressing the maximum dose tolerable to normal tissues and balancing it with an acceptable risk of morbidity. Traditionally, treatment has included irradiation of the whole pelvis followed by a boost dose to the prostate or prostate bed. Two plans dominate the national practice in the United States—the four-field technique (Fig. 3.8) and the bilateral 120° arcs.[45] Immobilization is important in minimizing the amount of normal tissues involved and results in a median error of 1 mm as compared to 3 mm in men who are not immobilized.[46]

With the advent of three-dimensional planning and conformal irradiation, it became feasible to deliver higher tumor doses to select targets and therefore improve tumor control probability while decreasing the morbidity.[1] This has resulted in an improved dose distribution with lower volumes of rectum and bladder within the high-dose volume as

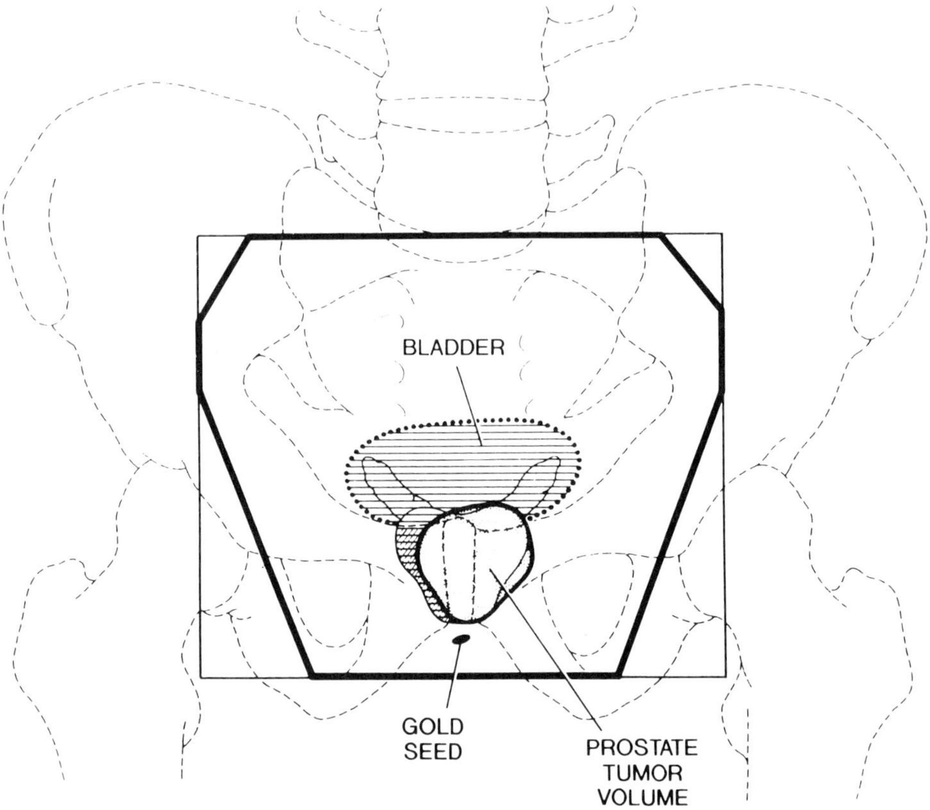

Fig. 3.8. Diagrammatic representation of the four-field "box" technique which utilizes anterior, posterior, right and left lateral radiation fields. A small pair of lateral fields may be used for a "boost" dose if a beam width improving device or compensator is used.[21]

compared with more conventional techniques. At the University of Chicago, a retrospective comparison of toxicities among groups treated with conventional, computed tomography (CT)-based manual planning, and beam's eye view based planning techniques[47] has shown that the beam's eye view technique resulted in the lowest toxicity. Three-dimensional planning has allowed tailoring of radiation fields to the precise shape of the target tissue and the conforming of the high-dose volume to structures felt to contain malignant cells while reducing the volume of bladder and rectum involved.[45]

At Memorial Sloan-Kettering Cancer Center conformal radiation was studied in 123 patients with localized prostate cancer. The dose was escalated from 64 to 66 to 70 to 75.6 Gy, and the 81 Gy arm has completed accrual.[48] Following this treatment, 99% of T1c to T2b patients had normalization of their PSA. Ninety percent of T2C patients and 81% of stage T3 patients also had their PSA decline to within the normal range. So far excellent acute tolerance has been noted up to 81 Gy with a median follow-up of 18 months.[4]

A prospective dose escalation trial performed at Michigan[49] used conformal planning and a six-field technique. Analysis found a dose–response relationship to local control

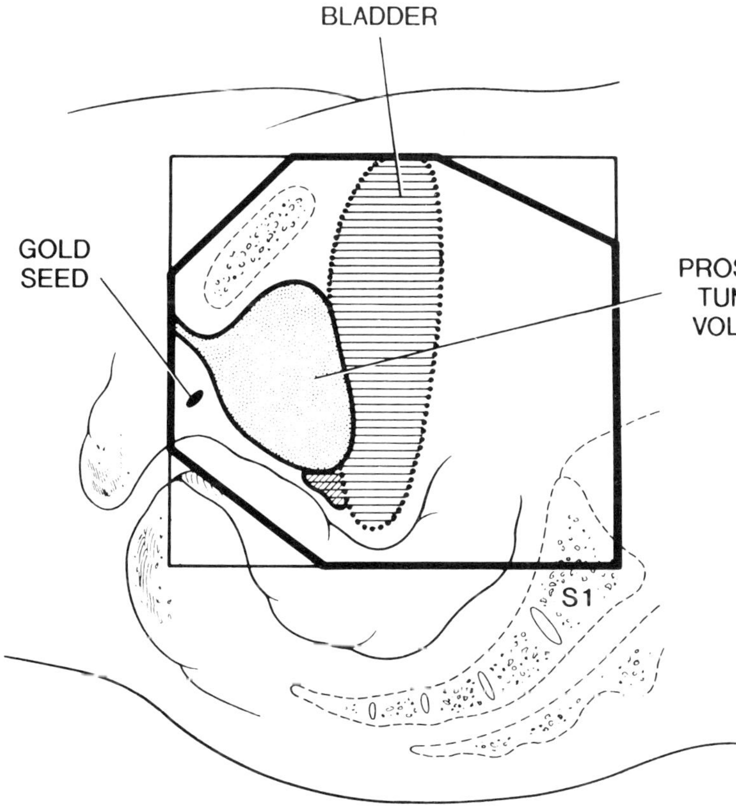

Fig. 3.8. Continued.

but also to complications. At the Fox Chase cancer center[46] conformal techniques have reduced the volume of the bladder and rectum included in the treatment field by an average of 14%.

Particle radiation therapy has also been explored in prostate cancer. The proton beam has unique physical characteristics that allow it to be shaped tightly to fit an irregular target volume without treating normal structures beyond that volume. It is the subject of ongoing study in at least two centers in the United States. The neutron is another particle whose biologic properties have been exploited. It has the potential biologic advantage over photons in killing slowly cycling cells or cells that are hypoxic. However, often there is similarly increased morbidity. The neutron therapy collaborative working group trial has randomized 182 patients with locally advanced or node positive prostate adenocarcinoma to compare photon treatment with neutron therapy. The neutron arm had an improved local control at 87% as compared with 68% in the photon arm. There was no improvement in overall survival. Significantly increased late complications were found in the neutron arm, which the authors attributed to inferior neutron beam shaping capabilities at certain institutions.[20] Particle therapy continues to evolve and may offer promising alternatives.

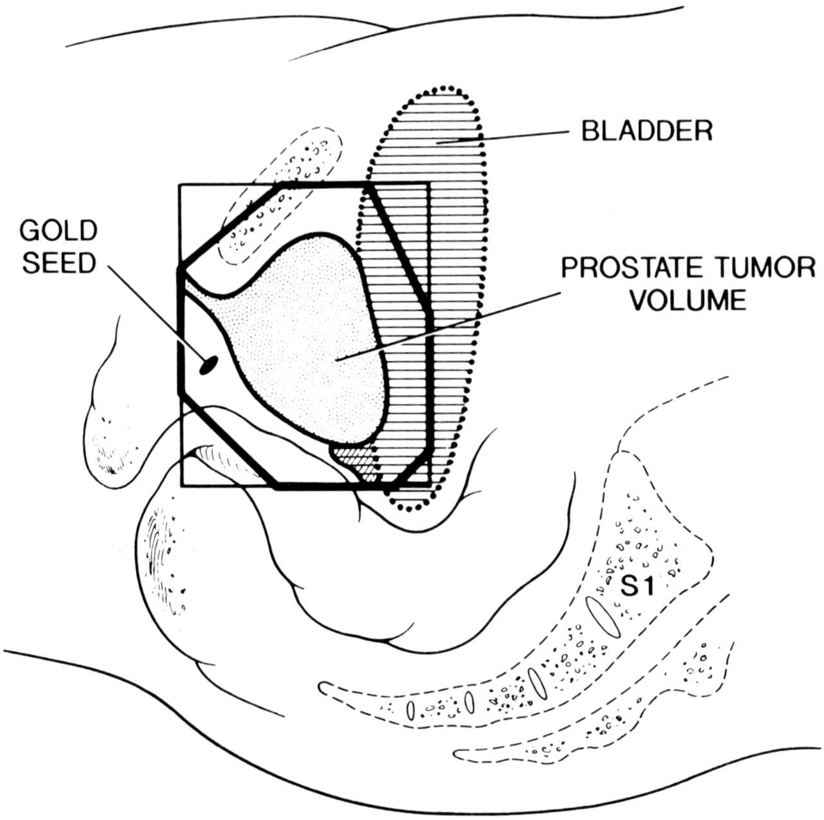

Fig. 3.8. Continued.

CONCLUSIONS

1. Conventional external beam radiation therapy produces high biochemical disease-free survival rates for patients with *true* early stage disease (T1–2a, Gleason $\leq$ 6, PSA $<$ 15 ng/ml).

2. The remainder of the T1–2 patients are unlikely to be cured and need more aggressive treatment. Whether this is best accomplished with conformal high-dose therapy or external beam in combination with androgen suppression remains uncertain.

3. T3–4 patients achieve high levels of durable clinical local control with conventional external beam radiation therapy but are very unlikely to be cured.

4. Neoadjuvant androgen suppression prior to external beam irradiation yields significantly higher local control and disease-free survival rates for T3–4 patients than radiation alone. Longer follow-up is required to ascertain whether or not this translates into increased cure rates.

5. Dose escalation and particle therapy hold promise in T3–4 disease but await mature modern trials.

6. External beam radiation may be used in an adjuvant setting to reduce local failure rates in men with positive surgical margins after radical prostatectomy. It may also be

used to salvage men with a rising PSA after surgery and a high probability of occult local failure.

REFERENCES

1. Perez CA, Hanks GE, Leibel SA, et al: Localized carcinoma of the prostate (stages T1b, T1c, T2, and T3). *Cancer* 72:3156–3173, 1993.
2. Willett CG, Zietman AL, Shipley WU, et al: The effect of pelvic radiation therapy on serum levels of prostate specific antigen. *J Urol* 151:1579–1581, 1994.
3. Kuban DA, El-Mahdi AM, Schellhammer PF: The significance of post irradiation prostate biopsy with long term follow up. *IJROBP* 24:409–414, 1993.
4. Leibel SA, Heiman R, Kutcher GJ, et al: Three dimensional conformal radiation therapy in locally advanced carcinoma of the prostate: preliminary results of a phase I dose escalation study. *IJROBP* 28:55–65, 1993.
5. Zietman AL, Shipley WU, Coen JJ: Radical prostatectomy and radical radiation therapy for clinical stages T1 to T2 adenocarcinoma of the prostate: new insights into outcome from repeat biopsy and PSA followup. *J Urol* 152:1806–1812, 1994.
6. Dugan TC, Shipley WU, Young RH, et al: Biopsy following external beam radiation therapy for adenocarcinoma of the prostate: correlation with original histologic grade and current PSA levels. *J Urol* 146:1313–1316, 1991.
7. Hanks GE, Krall JM, Hanlon AL, et al: Patterns of Care and RTOG studies in prostate cancer: long term survival, hazard rate observations, and possibilities of cure. *IJROBP* 28:39–45, 1994.
8. Hanks GE, Hanlon A, Schultheiss T, et al: Early prostate cancer: the national results of radiation treatment from the POC and RTOG studies with prospects for improvement with conformal radiation and adjuvant androgen deprivation. *J Urol* 152:1775–1780, 1994.
9. Lee RJ, Sause WT: Surgically staged patients with prostate carcinoma treated with definitive radiation therapy: 15 year results. *Urology* 43:640, 1994.
10. Schellhammer PF, El-Mahdi AM, Wright GL, et al: Prostate specific antigen to determine progression free survival after radiation therapy for localized carcinoma of the prostate. *Urology* 42:13, 1993.
11. Colvett KT, Zietman AL, Shipley WU: Radiation therapy for patients with T1 and T2a (B1) prostate cancer: selection yields high success rates maintained more than 10 years after treatment. In Khoury S, Murphy GP, Chatelaine C, et al (eds): *Proceedings of the 4th International Symposium on Recent Advances in Urologic Cancer*. Davis, Med Edition Pub., 1995, pp 214–220.
12. Bagshaw MA, Cox RS, Hancock SL: Control of prostate cancer with radiotherapy: long term results. *J Urol* 152:1781–1785, 1994.
13. Zagars GK, von Eschenbach AC, Ayala AG: Prognostic factors in prostate cancer. *Cancer* 72:1709–1725, 1993.
14. Stamey TA, Ferrari MK, Schmid HP: The value of serial prostate specific antigen determinations 5 years following radiotherapy: steeply increasing values characterize 80% of patients. *J Urol* 150:1856–1859, 1993.
15. Freiha FS: A comparative study of external beam irradiation teletherapy and radical retropubic prostatectomy in men with clinically localized prostate cancer and pathologically negative lymph nodes: 10 year follow up. In Khoury S, Murphy GP, Chatelain C, et al (eds): *Proceed-*

ings of the 4th International Symposium on Recent Advances in Urologic Cancer. Paris, Med. Edition Pub., 1995, pp 221–224.

16. Zietman AL, Coen JJ, Dallow KC, et al: The treatment of prostate cancer by conventional radiation therapy: an analysis of long-term outcome. *IJROBP* 32:287–292, 1995.
17. Bagshaw MA, Kaplan ID, Cox RC: Radiation therapy for localized disease. *Cancer* 71:939–952, 1993.
18. Perez CA, Lee HK, Georgiou A, et al: Technical and tumor-related factors affecting outcome of definitive irradiation for localized cancer of the prostate. *IJROBP* 26:581–591, 1993.
19. Russell KJ, Caplan RJ, Laramore GE, et al: Photon vs. fast neutron external beam radiotherapy in the treatment of locally advanced prostate cancer: results of a randomized trial. *IJROBP* 28:47–54, 1993.
20. Shipley WU, Verhey LJ, Munzenrider JE, et al: Advanced prostate cancer: the results of a randomized comparative trial of high dose irradiation boosting with conformal protons compared with conventional dose irradiation using photons alone. *IJROBP* 32:3–12, 1995.
21. Corn BW, Hanks GE, Schultheiss TE, et al: Conformal treatment of prostate cancer with improved targeting: superior prostate-specific antigen response compared to standard treatment. *IJROBP* 32:325–330, 1995.
22. Benk VA, Adams JA, Shipley WU, et al: Late rectal bleeding following combined x-ray and proton high dose irradiation for stages T3–T4 prostate cancer. *IJROBP* 26:551, 1993.
23. Pilepich MV, Krall JM, Al-Sarraf M, et al: Androgen deprivation with radiation therapy compared with radiation therapy alone for locally advanced prostate carcinoma: a RTOG randomized comparative trial. *Urology* 45:616–623, 1995.
24. Pilepich MV: Combined radiation therapy and endocrine therapy in locally advanced prostate cancer. In Vogelzang NJ, Scardino PT, Shipley WU, et al (eds): *Comprehensive Textbook of Genitourinary Oncology*. Baltimore, Williams and Wilkins (*In press*).
25. Pilepich MV, Caplan R, Byhardt RW, et al: Phase III trial of androgen suppression using goserelin in unfavorable prognostic carcinoma of the prostate treated with definitive radiation therapy (report of RTOG 85-31). Abstract 631. *Proc ASCO* 14:239, 1995.
26. Zietman AL, Shipley WU, Willett CG: Residual disease following radical surgery or radiation therapy for prostate cancer. *Cancer* 71:959–969, 1993.
27. Zietman AL: When should radiation therapy follow radical prostatectomy in the management of prostate cancer? *Mayo Clin Proc* 69:700, 1994.
28. Frazier HA, Robertson JE, Humphrey PA, et al: Is prostate specific antigen of clinical importance in evaluating outcome after radical prostatectomy? *J Urol* 149:516, 1993.
29. Epstein JI, Carmichael MJ, Pizor G, et al: Influence of capsular penetration on progression following radical prostatectomy: a study of 196 cases with long term follow up. *J Urol* 150:135, 1993.
30. Zietman AL: The role of radiation as adjuvant or salvage therapy following radical prostatectomy. In Vogelzang NJ, Scardino PT, Shipley WU, et al (eds): *Comprehensive Textbook of Genitourinary Oncology*. Baltimore, Williams and Wilkins (*In press*).
31. Link P, Freiha FS, Stamey TA: Adjuvant radiation therapy in patients with detectable prostate specific antigen following radical prostatectomy. *J Urol* 145:532, 1991.
32. Freeman JA, Lieskovsky G, Cook DW, et al: Radical retropubic prostatectomy and post-operative adjuvant radiation for pathological stage c (pCN0) prostate cancer from 1976–1989: intermediate findings. *J Urol* 149:1029, 1993.

33. Meier R, Mark R, St. Royal L, et al: Postoperative radiation therapy after radical prostatectomy for prostate carcinoma. *Cancer* 70:1960–1966, 1992.

34. McCarthy JF, Catalona WJ, Hudson MA: Effect of radiation therapy on detectable serum PSA levels following radical prostatectomy: early vs. delayed treatment. *J Urol* 151:1575–1578, 1994.

35. Zietman AL, Coen JJ, Shipley WU, et al: Adjuvant irradiation following radical prostatectomy for adenocarcinoma of the prostate: analysis of freedom from PSA failure. *Urology* 42:292, 1993.

36. Lange PH, Lighter DJ, Medini E, et al: The effect of radiation therapy after radical prostatectomy in patients with elevated prostate specific antigen levels. *J Urol* 144:927, 1990.

37. Hudson MA, Catalona WJ: Effect of adjuvant radiation therapy on prostate specific antigen following radical prostatectomy. *J Urol* 143:1174, 1990.

38. Schild SE, Wong WW, Grado GL, et al: Radiotherapy for isolated increases in serum PSA levels after radical prostatectomy. *Mayo Clin Proc* 69:613–619, 1994.

39. Shipley WU, Zietman AL, Hanks GE, et al: Treatment related sequelae following external beam radiation for prostate cancer: a review with an update in patients with stages T1 and T2 tumors. *J Urol* 152:1799, 1994.

40. Green N, Treible D, Wallack H: Prostate cancer: post-irradiation incontinence. *J Urol* 144:307–309, 1990.

41. Goldstein I, Feldman MI, Declose PJ, et al: Radiation associated impotence. *JAMA* 251:903, 1984.

42. Lawton CA, Won M, Pilepich MV, et al: Long term treatment sequelae following external beam irradiation for adenocarcinoma of the prostate: analysis of RTOG studies 7506 and 7706. *Int Radiat Oncol Biol Phys* 21:935, 1991.

43. Hanks GE, Martz KL, Diamond JJ: The effect of dose on local control of prostate cancer. *Int Radiat Oncol Biol Phys* 15:1299–1305, 1988.

44. Pilepich MV, Krall J, George FW: Treatment related morbidity in phase III RTOG studies of extended field irradiation for cancer of the prostate. *Int Radiat Oncol Biol Phys* 10:1861, 1984.

45. Epstein BE, Hanks GE: Radiation therapy techniques and dose selection in the treatment of prostate cancer. *Semin Rad Oncol* 3(3):179–186, 1993.

46. Soffen EM, Hanks GE, Hwang CC, et al: Conformal static field therapy for low volume low grade prostate cancer with rigid immobilization. *Int Radiat Oncol Biol Phys* 20:141–146, 1991.

47. Vijayakumor S, Awan A, Karrison T, et al: Acute toxicity during external beam radiotherapy for localized prostate cancer: comparison of different techniques. *Int Radiat Oncol Biol Phys* 25:359–371, 1993.

48. Leibel SA, Zelefsky MJ, Kutcher GJ, et al: Three dimensional conformal radiation therapy in localized carcinoma of the prostate: interim report of a phase I dose escalation study. *J Urol* 152:1792–1798, 1994.

49. Sandler HM, Perez-Tamayo C, Ten HR, et al: Dose escalation for Stage C (T3) prostate cancer: minimal rectal toxicity observed using conformal therapy. *Radiother Oncol* 23:53–54, 1992.

4

Radical Retropubic Prostatectomy Using Wide Excision (Non-Nerve-Sparing) or Nerve-Sparing Techniques: Improved Cancer Control vs. Potency Preservation

Robert A. Stephenson
Richard G. Middleton

Anatomic constraints severely limit the extent of excision of normal periprostatic tissues during radical prostatectomy. Not surprisingly, positive surgical margins are frequently noted (25–50% of cases) in contemporary radical prostatectomy series.[1–5] Partial or complete penetration of the prostate capsule is also frequently noted (approximately 60–80% of cases). Recent reports have documented the unfavorable impact of both positive margins and capsular penetration on progression-free survival.[1–3] This chapter reports on surgical methods which are performed with special attention paid to extending the margin of attached periprostatic tissue. These wide excision (non-nerve-sparing) surgical methods offer the potential to improve cancer control in patients who elect a more extensive surgical approach.

Over the last 10 years radical prostatectomy has undergone a resurgence in popularity. This resurgence has been concurrent with the advent of now widely practiced nerve sparing surgical modifications which offer the preservation of potency in a majority of selected patients.[6] However, the already limited extent of excision in radical prostatectomy can be limited further by nerve sparing techniques. This is because these techniques are designed to dissect close to the prostatic surface in order to preserve the neurovascular bundles and potency. It is of particular importance that capsular penetration is anatomically most common in the posterolateral region of the prostatic hilum (the region of the neurovascular bundle).[7,8] For this reason there is a potential increased risk of incomplete excision when nerve-sparing procedures are used. Since the introduction of nerve-sparing techniques, Walsh and others have consistently cautioned against using nerve sparing techniques in patients suspected of extraprostatic disease.[9,10] While the experience of many groups with nerve-sparing techniques are reported in the literature, little has been published regarding systematic surgical approaches to widely excise all available periprostatic tissues, nor have issues regarding selection of nerve-sparing versus wide excision approaches for individual patients been adequately addressed. We will attempt to address these issues in the sections that follow.

NERVE-SPARING RADICAL RETROPUBIC PROSTATECTOMY

The history and surgical technique of nerve-sparing radical retropubic prostatectomy have been well described in the literature. It is important to note that there are two surgical methods described for nerve-sparing radical prostatectomy. Walsh first described potency preservation using a retrograde (distal to proximal) dissection, where apical division and prostate mobilization occur concurrent with nerve-sparing dissection.[6] The group at Stanford University describe a technique where the neurovascular bundles are dissected free from the prostate prior to division of the urethra and mobilization of the prostate.[11] Using these techniques, good but not uniformly superior cancer control rates have been documented for individuals with organ-confined pathology.[2,3] Poor cancer control outcomes in organ-confined cases are presumably due to either pathologically unrecognized and incompletely excised local disease or to undetectable micrometastatic disease. Results in cases with extraprostatic extension or positive margins, frequent occurrences in most surgical case populations, as expected, have poorer outcomes for similar reasons.

Reported postoperative potency rates after nerve-sparing radical prostatectomy have been related to age, with approximately 70–80% preservation of potency for men in their 50s, 50% preservation for men in their 60s, and 30% preservation for men in their 70s.[10] Rigorous assessment of postoperative potency with respect to rigidity of erections, duration of erections, and need for the use of adjunctive methods for relative degrees of postoperative erectile dysfunction have not been reported in the literature. Further, frequency and quality of sexual intercourse before and after surgery or other global measures of the impact of therapy on sexual function have not been accurately assessed. Studies of these quality issues are important in order for physicians and patients to balance decisions regarding nerve-sparing and wide excision radical prostatectomy.

WIDE EXCISION (NON-NERVE-SPARING) RADICAL RETROPUBIC PROSTATECTOMY

In order to perform an optimal wide excision radical prostatectomy, it is important that the surgeon understand the central problem of sheer forces. During a radical prostatectomy, significant sheer forces occur once the urethra is divided at the apex. These forces tend to strip away attached periprostatic tissues during anterior retraction of the prostatic apex, and during mobilization of the posterior prostatic surface. An excellent method to avoid the unwanted effect of these sheer forces is to release the posterior periprostatic tissues from their nonprostatic attachments *prior* to division of the puboprostatic ligaments and urethra. This is done by first performing a perirectal dissection, posterior and lateral to the prostate, in order to release the periprostatic tissues from their posterior attachments, while leaving them freely attached to the prostate and thereby protected from subsequent sheer forces. A description of the technique of wide excision radical prostatectomy follows.

Surgical Technique

A priori perirectal dissection is performed prior to division of the puboprostatic ligaments. Complete opening of the endopelvic fascia is performed. Incomplete opening of this fascia, in particular posteriorly, will result in inadequate lateral mobility of the prostate and poor visualization during the perirectal dissection. Lateral displacement of the prostate reveals a glistening fascial covering overlying the rectal surface (Fig. 4.1). At this rectal surface there are two or three fascial layers with intervening fat. Beginning

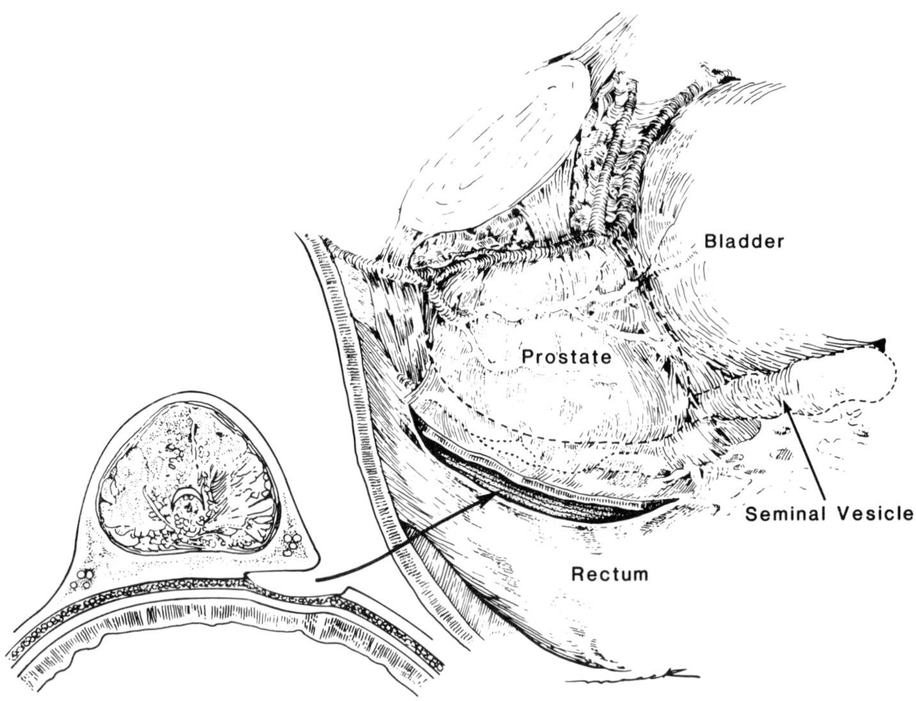

Fig. 4.1. A priori perirectal incision. This incision is made through two or three delicate fascial layers with intervening fat. When made properly the longitudinal fibers of the rectum should be directly visualized at the base of the incision. The incision is made from base to apex, 1–2 cm lateral and posterior to the prostate.

near the prostatic base, these layers are divided over a presenting right angle with cautery or Metzenbaum scissors. The line of dissection moves from prostatic base to apex approximately 1.0–1.5 cm lateral and posterior to the prostate directly on the rectal surface (Figure 4.1). Perirectal dissection is complete when the longitudinal fibers of the rectum are seen between the two leaflets of the incision and when a finger within this incision palpates the posterior apical urethral junction without bridging perirectal fascial layers or rectourethralis musculature. The releasing effect of this perirectal incision assures that the tissues of the anterior leaflet of the perirectal incision (the posterolateral periprostatic tissues) are left attached to the prostate, yet are free from all other attachments and, therefore, will not later be stripped away after urethral division, or during the sheer forces which take place while freeing the posterior prostatic surface.

At this point the puboprostatic ligaments, dorsal vein complex, urethra, and Denonvilliers plate are divided at the level of the prostatic apex, taking care to leave an adequate urethral margin. At the level of the apical–urethral junction, the posterolateral periprostatic tissues (neurovascular bundle, etc.) are divided at right angle to the urethral axis. This is done by inserting a right angle into the perirectal incision immediately anterior to the rectum (the rectum is directly visualized in the incision) in order to present the posterolateral periprostatic tissues for division with scissors or electrocautery.

Dissection within the perirectal pocket and directly on the longitudinal fibers of the rectum assures removal of all layers of Denonvilliers fascia together with all available periprostatic tissues. This is important to avoid incomplete resection of tumor along the posterior surface of the prostate as described by Villers et al.[12] The perirectal incision gives access to multiple potential points of dissection along the longitudinal fibers of the rectum. This option, to select from a variety of dissection points, is particularly useful when the rectum is firmly adherent to the prostate at a specific site. In this situation, another site of dissection can then be selected, allowing the adherent site to be dissected more safely at a subsequent time in the procedure. The perirectal dissection as just described can be performed in conjunction with either retrograde (Walsh technique) or antegrade (Campbell technique) surgical approaches. The modification adds approximately 10 minutes to the procedure. It can be performed while waiting for the frozen section results of the lymph node dissection.

Using the retrograde approach (Walsh), the plane of dissection directly on the longitudinal rectal fibers is continued from distal to proximal all the way to the tip of the seminal vesicles in order to allow complete excision of the seminal vesicles with their fatty and fascial coverings. The seminal vesicles should be encased in these coverings at the conclusion of the procedure. The vascular pedicles to the prostate and seminal vesicles should be divided just proximal to the tips of each seminal vesicle. This can be performed at this stage in the procedure or later, after the plane between posterior bladder wall and the anterior surface of the seminal vesicles has been defined.

Figure 4.2 shows the extent of excised periprostatic that remains with the prostate on transverse sections from the prostatic base to apex when wide excision methods are used. While Fig. 4.2 is an example of bilateral wide excision specimens, the procedure can be performed unilaterally with contralateral nerve sparing. As with bilateral wide excision procedures, unilateral nerve-sparing procedures should also be performed with a posterior dissection directly on the longitudinal fibers of the rectum in order to remove all layers of Denonvilliers fascia and minimize the risk of posterior positive margins.[12]

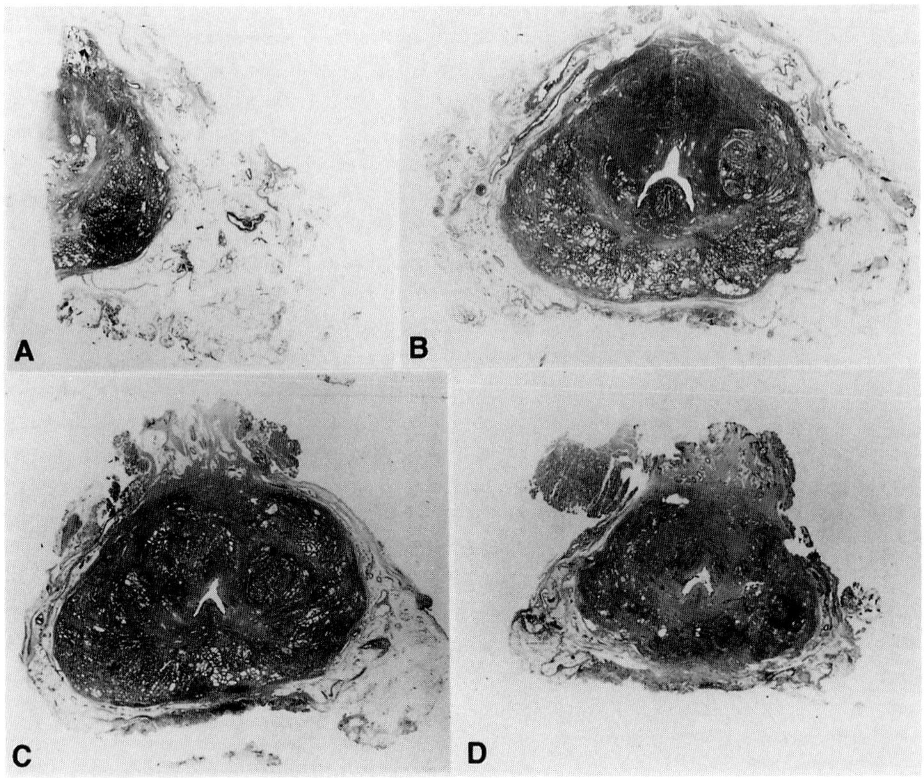

Fig. 4.2. Photographs of transverse whole organ sections of a wide excision radical prostatectomy. Note the quantities of excised periprostatic tissue. **A:** Prostatic base (specimen bivalved); **B** and **C:** sections of mid prostate; **D:** apical.

WIDE EXCISION VS. NERVE-SPARING RADICAL PROSTATECTOMY: ISSUES FOR DISCUSSION

The object of this chapter is to raise the following question: Is there a systematic method by which the excision of all possible periprostatic tissues may be performed and thereby offer patients improved cancer surgery and improved survival? No currently available information answers this question directly or unequivocally. However, it is a generally accepted surgical dictum that wide margins will improve surgical results. Further, it is important to note that metastasis research in a variety of tumor systems shows that cells with aggressive biologic phenotypes will demonstrate their phenotype by their location.[13] In other words, tumor progression and metastasis are not random events. Tumor cells reach a given location by virtue of cellular characteristics of individual cells that have enabled them to arrive and function at that location. These characteristics of cellular aggressiveness are less likely to be noted in tumor cells of the primary tumor. In prostate cancer, Mohler et al. have noted that nuclear shape analysis, a measure of biologic aggressiveness, is related to tumor cell location.[14] They observed that cells in periprostatic adipose tissue and in lymph nodes have more aggressive nuclear shape characteristics than tumor cells within the prostate. Cells on the outer edge of a primary tumor within the prostate also have more aggressive nuclear shape characteristics than those at the center of the tumor. The group from Stanford University have shown prostate specific antigen (PSA) data in support of this general concept by noting that residual cells in patients after radical prostatectomy, with PSA defined failure, have substantially higher PSA doubling times, another measure of biologic aggressiveness, than do the cells of primary tumors (reflected in the preoperative PSA doubling times).[15] Partin et al. showed a significant difference in disease-free survival in patients with "established" capsular penetration who underwent excision of at least one neurovascular bundle versus those undergoing bilateral nerve preservation.[16] The observations listed above appear to indicate that it is important to attempt removal of these potentially more malignant cells using optimal wide excision surgical techniques whenever possible.

Villers et al. and Rosen et al. have reported the most common site of prostate cancer capsular penetration is in the posterolateral region, the region of the neurovascular bundle.[7,8] This observation suggests that the posterolateral and adjoining periprostatic regions may be at increased risk of incomplete excision during nerve-sparing surgery. As stated earlier, Walsh and others have been careful to emphasize that nerve-sparing radical prostatectomy holds the potential for incomplete excision of pericapsular disease, and should be avoided in cases where capsular penetration is likely.[9] In view of the frequency of capsular penetration, it is conceptually appealing to consider a systematic method of wide excision where removal of all available periprostatic tissue may offer cancer control benefits to patients with carcinoma of the prostate. While wide excision surgical methods will result in loss of potency, intracorporal injection, vacuum devices, and prosthetic implants offer suitable means for achieving sexual activity after radical prostatectomy.

Clinically relevant questions include: Will cancer control indeed be improved using optimal surgical methods and in what fraction of patients? To whom should wide excision radical prostatectomy be offered? How are patients who may benefit to be selected? How do patients and physicians weigh the relative benefits, risks, and disadvantages of the important quality of life issue of potency against improved cancer control and survival?

Based on our experience with 53 cases of wide excision radical prostatectomy, we believe that positive margin rates can be reduced using a priori perirectal dissection techniques as outlined earlier in this chapter.[17] Positive margin rates of 13% were observed in this series. These results compare favorably with the 25–50% margin positive rates in comparable series where wide excision techniques were not exclusively used. Clinical stage was approximately 20% T1b/T1c and 80% T2 in this series. Pathologic staging was based on whole organ mounts at 3–4 mm intervals. Approximately 45% of cases were non-organ-confined.

In general, if a surgical method is going to improve cancer control, reduction of positive margin rates should be observed. While a positive margin rate is the most immediate method for determining completeness of excision, it is rather insensitive as a predictor of final outcome. Observations over time including local recurrence, rising PSA, disease progression, and survival are better parameters for assessing the adequacy of surgical therapy. Adequate long-term measures of outcome are currently unavailable in this series. However, postoperative PSA monitoring in these patients shows undetectable PSAs in all patients with the exception of one patient with minimal seminal vesicle involvement and negative margin of resection whose latest PSA is 0.4 ng/ml (preoperative PSA 65, follow-up—138 weeks). Median overall follow-up for this series was 120 weeks (range 64–195 weeks).

We believe it is important for urologists to carefully evaluate issues of potency and cancer control as they relate to nerve sparing and wide excision radical prostatectomy. Further, it is important for urologists to be facile with both of these surgical techniques. In addition, patients need to be educated regarding the issues of potency and cancer control, as well as the unavoidable uncertainties of treatment selection, in order to make treatment decisions that are in keeping with these issues, and with the patients' own values and priorities.

REFERENCES

1. Paulson DF, Moul JW, Walther PJ: Radical prostatectomy for clinical stage T1-2N0M0 prostatic adenocarcinoma: long-term results. *J Urol* 144:1180–1184, 1990.
2. Epstein JI, Pizov G, Walsh PC: Correlation of pathologic findings with progression after radical retropubic prostatectomy. *Cancer* 71:3582–3593, 1993.
3. Morton RA, Steiner MS, Walsh PC: Cancer control following anatomical radical prostatectomy: an interim report. *J Urol* 145:1197–1200, 1991.
4. Epstein JI, Carmichael M, Partin AW, et al: Is tumor volume an independent predictor of progression following radical prostatectomy? A multivariate analysis of 185 clinical stage B adenocarcinomas of the prostate with 5 years of follow-up. *J Urol* 149:1478–1481, 1993.
5. Stamey TA, Villers A, McNeal JE, et al: Positive surgical margins at radical prostatectomy: importance of the apical dissection. *J Urol* 143:1166–1173, 1990.
6. Eggleston JC, Walsh PC: Radical prostatectomy with preservation of sexual function: pathological findings in the first 100 cases. *J Urol* 134:1146–1148, 1985.
7. Villers A, McNeal JE, Redwine EA, et al: The role of perineural space invasion in the local spread of prostatic adenocarcinoma. *J Urol* 142:763–768, 1989.
8. Rosen MA, Goldstone L, Lapin S, et al: Frequency and location of extracapsular extension and positive margins in radical prostatectomy specimens. *J Urol* 148:331–337, 1992.
9. Walsh PC: Radical retropubic prostatectomy. In Walsh PC, Retik AB, Stamey TA, et al (eds): *Campbell's Urology*, ed 6. Philadelphia, WB Saunders, 1992, vol 3, sect XIV, chap 28, p 2865.
10. Walsh PC: Radical prostatectomy, preservation of sexual function, cancer control: the controversy. *Urol Clin North Am* 14:663–673, 1987.
11. Freiha FS: Radical retropubic prostatectomy. In Crawford ED, Das S (eds): *Cancer of the Prostate*. New York, Marcel Dekker, 1993, pp 189–223.
12. Villers A, McNeal JE, Freiha FS, et al: Invasion of Denonvilliers' fascia in radical prostatectomy specimens. *J Urol* 149:793–798, 1993.
13. Fidler IJ: Critical factors in the biology of human cancer metastasis: Twenty-eighth G. H. A. Clowes Memorial Award Lecture. *Cancer Res* 50:6130–6138, 1990.
14. Mohler JL, Figlesthaler WM, Zhang XZ, et al: Nuclear shape analysis for the assessment of local invasion and metastases in clinically localized prostate carcinoma. *Cancer* 74:1996–3001, 1994.
15. Schmid HP, McNeal JE, Stamey TA: Observations on the doubling time of prostate cancer. The use of serial prostate specific antigen in patients with untreated disease as a measure of increasing cancer volume. *Cancer* 71:2031–2040, 1993.

16. Partin AW, Borland RN, Epstein JI, et al: Influence of wide excision of the neurovascular bundle(s) on the prognosis in men with clinically localized prostate cancer with established capsular penetration. *J Urol* 150:142–148, 1993.
17. Stephenson RA, Middleton RG: Reduction in the rate of positive surgical margins for clinically localized prostate cancer—technique and results of apriori per-rectal dissection in non-nerve sparing radical retropubic prostatectomy. *J Urol* 151:256A, 1994.

5

Treatment of the Patient with a Rising PSA (Biochemical Failure) Following Radical Prostatectomy

Richard A. Santucci
Paul H. Lange

As radical prostatectomy (RP) has increasingly become the treatment of choice for stage B prostate cancer, there are expanding numbers of patients with potentially persistent disease after this treatment who might benefit from adjuvant therapies. This stems mostly from the fact that preoperative staging is inaccurate, and up to 50% of these patients will not have organ-confined disease after RP.[1,2]

A popular form of adjuvant therapy for these patients has been local radiation. This is because although it has never been proven to prolong life, it seems to decrease the incidence and severity of local recurrence. Local radiation causes significant and, in some cases, durable decreases in circulating prostate specific antigen (PSA), which may reflect its potent antitumor effect. These observations, and the fact that it can be performed with few complications, make it an attractive option in those cases where RP has not cured the patient.

In this article, we will first review the pathologic and operative features that affect persistence rates after radical prostatectomy. Then, we will discuss the methods of detecting disease persistence after this surgery, including digital rectal examination (DRE), PSA, ultrasensitive PSA, ultrasound, and needle biopsy. Finally, we will discuss in detail the value of adjuvant radiation, as well as touch upon other treatments such as antiandrogens and chemotherapy.

CANCER PERSISTENCE RATES AFTER RADICAL PROSTATECTOMY

A variety of methods and terminologies are used to describe persistent disease after radical prostatectomy, most of which yield a figure around 50%. Some researchers have used cancer-free survival after RP as the best measure of cancer persistence. This number is reported to be as low as 33%,[3] while others place it closer to 50%[4,5] to 66%.[6–8] The ideal follow-up of these patients, rarely attained, is thought to be 15 years, though recurrences as long as 20 years out have been reported.[9] The pattern of failure after RP is biased toward metastatic disease, with half or more presenting with distant tumor spread.[1,2,4,10]

As expected, cancer persistence rates after RP are related to the preoperative clinical stage. Local failure rates are lowest with B1 disease (11%), higher with B2 disease (18%), and highest for C disease (31%).[4] Because the accuracy of preoperative staging is not ideal, this relationship is not perfect. Carter et al. found that almost half of the preoperative A2 or B patients really had C or D1 disease, thus making even this predictor tenuous.[11]

Cancer persistence after RP has also been demonstrated by autopsy studies[10] and postoperative detection of circulating PSA. Use of PSA in recent years has improved the detection rate of recurrent prostate cancer, and thus modern series tend toward higher estimations of persistence. An example of this is found in a recent study by Partin et al.[12] which defined persistence not as clinically evident local disease or metastases (as the older studies had), but as a detectable PSA. They showed persistence of disease in up to three-fourths of patients with aggressive tumors (capsular penetration) by 4 years.

Parenthetically, the reader must remember that the term "recurrence" is only a euphemism for "persistence" of disease. These terms, however, are used interchangeably in the literature and throughout this article.

THE EFFECT OF PATHOLOGIC FEATURES ON TUMOR RECURRENCE

It is important to understand the definitions and consequences of post-RP pathologic characteristics. These factors will affect not only the rate of disease persistence, but can also be used to select those patients who might benefit from adjuvant therapy in the absence of the signs of tumor recurrence. The classical features are capsular penetration, surgical margins, and extraprostatic extension of cancer, particularly to the seminal vesicles.

Capsular Penetration

Few pathologic issues in prostate cancer are as divisive as the question of the effect of capsular penetration on the rate of tumor recurrence. Most studies have found no negative effects of capsular penetration. Specifically, they found no correlation to subsequent failure[2,4,13–16] or patient survival.[4,9,13,16] In fact, Stamey et al. found no correlation between capsular penetration and any other pathologic adverse feature such as tumor size, seminal vesicle invasion, or positive lymph nodes.[15]

Others have argued that capsular penetration predicts a high risk of failure, either because it is associated with positive margins, or because it is correlated with increased tumor aggressivity in general. For example, McNeal et al. found that capsular penetration *is* correlated with cancer volume and positive nodes.[17] Others have found a higher risk of persistent disease,[14] decreased patient survival,[1] and a shorter time to detectable recurrence with capsular penetration.[9]

In summary, capsular penetration may be a difficult parameter to study, as even skilled pathologists find it problematic to define.[14] As we have described, opinions regarding its importance vary widely. Consequently, capsular penetration should probably not be used as a parameter to suggest the need for adjuvant therapy in the absence of other indications of disease persistence such as PSA.

Positive Margins

Although it seems axiomatic that positive margins would be an invariable predictor of persistent disease, opinions vary as to its prognostic significance. Some researchers have found it predictive of failure, leading to almost twice the recurrence rates of organ-confined disease.[14] However, in these studies persistence rates were not 100%, indicating that positive margins do not predict eventual cancer recurrence in all cases. In fact, others have argued that the presence of cancer cells at the surgical margin does not mean that tumor has been left behind. In one study of over 1,000 radical prostatectomies, positive margins were not significant in predicting progression or survival.[18] Furthermore, Epstein analyzed the neurovascular bundles of 40 patients who first had a nerve-sparing prostatectomy, then had the bundles resected because of fear of local spread in that area. Fully 28% of these cases had tumor extending to the inked margins of resection, but actually had no further cancer found in the surrounding tissue.[19]

Tumor Volume

Tumor volume is also a controversial subject. Epstein et al. found tumor volume predicted progression, although not as well as Gleason score or surgical margins.[8] They found that tumors averaging 2.4 cc did not usually progress, while those over 4.3 cc did progress.[8] In general, the weight of evidence suggests that tumor volume is a good, but certainly not the best, predictor of tumor persistence after RP.

The percentage of the prostate that is involved with cancer is very much like the tumor volume. Epstein et al.[8] found that in general, patients with a small percentage of the prostate involved with tumor (7%) had less chance of progression after RP than those with higher percentage of cancer. However, there was a wide distribution and many patients did not adhere to this rule. Frazier et al.[2] found a much higher cutoff of 25% involvement, over which there was a significantly greater chance of biochemical failure after RP.

Gleason Score

Gleason score has been called the prognostic factor with the most consistent correlation to poor outcome.[18] It is highly correlated with recurrence[2,6,8,14,18–20,21] and survival.[9] The cutoff appears to cluster around a Gleason score of 7 or 8, above which 5-year survival plummets to a third of that in lower grade tumors.[9] As with all the pathologic parameters studies, some have also found Gleason score to have no relation to subsequent poor outcome.[22]

Seminal Vesicle Invasion

The ominous nature of seminal vesicle invasion is well recognized. It bodes a threefold higher chance of postoperative biochemical failure,[2] predicting both increased local failure[6,16] and metastatic disease.[6,16,18] Even after adjuvant radiotherapy, 5-year cancer recurrence rates were doubled in patients who had seminal vesicle invasion.[23]

Ploidy

Ploidy has only recently been studied as an independent predictor of recurrence after RP. Morgan et al.[7] found that aneuploid tumors had a threefold greater risk of recurrence than diploid tumors. Early biochemical failure was almost twice as likely in the aneuploid group, and aneuploidy ultimately predicted poorer disease-specific survival for those patients. Carmichael et al.[21] found ploidy to be useful in predicting failure in a small subset of patients who had low Gleason score and yet still developed persistent disease after RP. Nonetheless, it is somewhat surprising that more confirmatory studies on this issue have not come forth. Accordingly, we believe it is still uncertain if ploidy is a significant independent predictor of tumor behavior.

THE EFFECT OF OPERATIVE FEATURES ON TUMOR RECURRENCE

Although most of the features of prostate cancer that predict poor outcomes are determined by the aggressivity of the tumor, some are determined by the surgeon. The surgeon may choose to excise wide margins or to save the nerves to the penis.

Effect of Nerve Sparing

The conventional wisdom is that nerve sparing does not increase the risk of leaving behind tumor when used on those patients with smaller tumors, or on the side not involved with tumor. Nerve sparing was actually associated with *lower* rates of positive surgical margins (45% compared with 58%) than non-nerve-sparing prostatectomies in a recent study.[9] Of course this bias occurs because nerve sparing is only offered to patients without suspicious or indurated margins, who naturally should have lower rates of extraprostatic spread. We do not really know the effect nerve sparing will have on long-term persistence rates, however if it is used indiscriminately, it will surely have a deleterious effect.

Wide Margins

An intriguing strategy in prostatectomy is to attempt to decrease the incidence of positive margins by excising as much tissue around the prostate as possible. This technique was favored in the early 1970s, and fell into disuse in the modern age of the Walsh anatomic prostatectomy and nerve sparing. Recent work by Stephenson and Middleton suggests that wide margins may dramatically reduce the incidence of positive surgical margins, from 50% to 13%.[24] Despite this, even wider excision of the prostate via exenteration or cystoprostatectomy has also been used in the face of advanced local disease with unencouraging results.[26]

THE DETECTION OF TUMOR RECURRENCE AFTER RADICAL PROSTATECTOMY

In the past, prostate cancer recurrence was detectable only by the crude signs of induration on digital rectal examination and obvious metastatic spread late in the course of disease. Recent years have seen an explosion in the tools used to detect persistent disease, including PSA, transrectal ultrasound (TRUS), and TRUS-guided anastomotic biopsies.

Digital Rectal Examination

DRE is often inadequate in the detection of local recurrence after RP. Up to 55% of those with biopsy-proven local recurrence will have a normal DRE.[22,27,28,29] After adjuvant treatment of recurrence with external beam radiation therapy (XRT), the DRE becomes even less diagnostic as nearly all patients get a hard smooth prostatic fossa which makes examination of cancer masses difficult. However, not everyone has found DRE inadequate after RP: Abi-Aad showed that 4 of 4 of his patients with positive anastamotic biopsy had an abnormal DRE,[30] and Parra showed that 15 of 20 of his biopsy-positive patients had one.[29] Probably, the interpretation of DRE is strongly dependent on examiner sensitivity and possibly foreknowledge of the patient's serum PSA level.

Prostatic Specific Antigen

Although evidence for the secretion of PSA from some nonprostatic tissue exists,[31–34] for practical purposes circulating PSA is not found after radical prostatectomy in the absence of cancer recurrence. In general, 100% of those with documented recurrence will have a detectable PSA.[15,35] Likewise, the absence of PSA after RP correlates well to the absence of persistent disease in over 90% of patients.[36] Undetectable PSA must be viewed with caution because some patients have a very small volume of persistent cancer and their PSA may take years to rise into the detectable (0.4 ng/ml) range.[36] In fact, late PSA failures up to 4½ years after RP have been reported.[37] Finally, some neuroendocrine prostate cancers will not secrete PSA despite bulky recurrence.[34]

Postoperative PSA predates clinically detectable cancer recurrence by more than a year, and is probably three times more sensitive than clinical examination.[2] PSA after RP is so specific that the early biochemical (PSA) failure rate predicts the late clinical failure rate exactly.[2] Of those who have detectable PSA after RP, a third do so by 6 months, 85% do so by 24 months, and nearly all do so by 36 months.[37]

PSA after RP might be able to do more than just detect recurrence. Danella et al.[37] found that PSA velocity after RP may delineate between metastatic spread and local recurrence. Patients with slow PSA doubling times had mostly local recurrence, while those with faster doubling times (>5 months) had mostly distant metastases. Partin et al.[12]

agree with this, but indicated that PSA velocity was best used in conjunction with other parameters. Finally, patients with initially detectable levels of PSA after RP often soon present with metastatic disease.[38]

The issue of retained benign prostatic hyperplasia (BPH) in the prostatic bed could theoretically confuse the picture of post-RP PSA. There is between a 6%[39] and 18%[22] incidence of residual BPH on needle biopsy in patients with elevated PSA after RP. However, two-thirds of these patients will eventually be discovered to have residual prostate cancer in the bed.[22,40] Accordingly, the finding of BPH nodule on anastomotic biopsies after RP should prompt a second biopsy, and even a third biopsy if PSA continues to rise. BPH should be considered the definitive diagnosis only in those patients with stable or very slowly rising PSA, after multiple biopsies.

More Sensitive PSA Bioassays

In the past, most of the PSA assays use a lower limit of detection of 0.4 ng/ml. Newer PSA assays allow detection of PSA to a limit of 0.1 ng/ml, which should increase its sensitivity in detecting persistent cancer. Use of this "micro" PSA technique has improved detection lead time over the standard by 1 year.[38,41] In our hands, at 8 months after RP, micro-PSA levels detected one-third more persistent cancers than the standard assays. All patients with a detectable micro-PSA had persistently elevated levels, and it sometimes took years to go from 0.1 ng/ml to the 0.4 ng/ml detected by the standard PSA assay.

More recently, even more sensitive "ultrasensitive" PSA assays have been created with the ability to detect PSA in the 0.01–0.04 ng/ml range and are being tested. These techniques promise to allow earlier adjuvant treatment of persistent prostate cancer. Perhaps more importantly, they might reduce the need to guess which patients might have a recurrence after RP by their pathologic features alone.

Even if the PSA detection threshold is pushed to the limit, there will always be those who initially have undetectable levels but later have a recurrence. To detect these patients, the technique of androgen provocative testing has been suggested by Lightner et al.[27] This would entail the temporary administration of exogenous testosterone in order to provoke detectable PSA levels in those with very small-volume persistent disease. This technique is currently being investigated in experimental models (P. H. Lange, unpublished data).

Transrectal Ultrasound

Ultrasound examination of the prostatic fossa after RP is difficult, and probably does not yield useful information. Up to 80% of patients felt to be clinically and biochemically free of disease have an anterior hypoechoic soft-tissue lesion which might be confused with carcinoma,[42] and 40% of known locally recurrent cancers have a normal TRUS,[30] yielding dismal performance characteristics. The only reliable TRUS sign of cancer recurrence seems to be a slight increase in the mean volume of perianastomotic tissue.[28] Otherwise, there is no consistent appearance of known recurrent tumors on TRUS; for example, half are isoechoic and half are hypoechoic.[30] Despite these limitations, some researchers have had success with TRUS after RP. Parra et al. felt that TRUS visualized pelvic recurrence in 19 of 20 biopsy-proven tumors. Seventy-two percent of these lesions were hypoechoic, and the rest were isoechoic.[29] Foster et al. found 95% correlation between a hypoechoic lesion near the anastomosis and subsequent positive biopsies in patients with elevated PSA after RP.[40] Despite these isolated successes, the best use of TRUS appears to be in the postoperative period, to guide biopsies of the prostatic fossa in cases of suspected recurrence based upon detectable PSA levels.

Random Needle Biopsy

Just as with the detection of primary prostate cancer, the first anastomotic biopsies were performed randomly, without TRUS guidance. Although it has been supplanted by TRUS-guided biopsy, random needle anastomotic biopsies taught us much about the incidence and detection of persistent disease after RP. Lightner et al. first proved that random anastomotic biopsy could detect persistent cancer in the face of negative computed tomography scans, bone scans, and cystoscopy studies.[27] These early random biopsies also help confirm the utility of post-RP PSA measurements by demonstrating a high rate of positive biopsies in those with detectable PSA after RP,[27,43] but a 0% rate of positive biopsies when the PSA was undetectable.[27]

Despite the fact that random biopsies were detecting between 40% and 60% of persistent cancer after RP, it became clear that they were not detecting 100% of the persistent tumors. Studies by Foster[40] showed that repeat random biopsies were often positive after an initial negative sampling. In fact, in patients who eventually had a positive anastomotic biopsy, 33% were diagnosed on the second or third biopsy.[40] The interval from RP to biopsy did not seem to affect the rate at which persistent disease was detected, with a range of 6 to 240 months.[40]

Transrectal Ultrasound-Guided Biopsy

Just as with the initial detection of prostate cancer, TRUS-guided anastomotic biopsies superseded random biopsies. Although TRUS itself could not identify cancer well, it could be used to guide the biopsy needle toward suspicious areas or masses. Despite this, TRUS-guided biopsies did not dramatically improve the rate of detection of persistent cancer, which remained about 50%.[22,44] The complication rate of this procedure is not widely described, although one study found gross hematuria in 5% after TRUS-guided biopsy.[44]

EXTERNAL BEAM RADIATION IN THE TREATMENT OF PERSISTENT CANCER FOLLOWING RADICAL PROSTATECTOMY

Before the advent of PSA testing, studies of adjuvant radiation therapy (ART) relied on the insensitive DRE to detect recurrence. Therefore, these studies will be favorably skewed for two reasons: (1) some disease-free patients were undoubtedly treated, and (2) some recurrences were not detected during the follow-up period. Therefore, any discussion of the merits of ART are best broken up into the pre- and post-PSA studies, since PSA allows a much more reliable method of detection and monitoring of persistent prostate cancer.

Adjuvant Radiation Therapy in the Pre-PSA Era

Caution must be exercised in interpreting data before the age of PSA. Some pre-PSA studies assert that local control is improved after ART,[45,46] however this may only indicate that radiotherapy only makes the DRE a less sensitive test. In fact, biopsy-proven persistent cancer after both primary radiation[22,44] and adjuvant radiation therapy is high, approaching 100% in some series.[47] It also occurs after adjuvant therapy even in those with unremarkable DRE.

If ART really does provide local control as some have asserted, it is unknown if this decreases later metastatic spread. It certainly does not seem to improve survival. In patients with pathologic C disease after RP, for example, several studies have shown no survival advantage of ART over surgery alone.[20,45,48–50]

Adjuvant Radiation Therapy in the Post-PSA Era

It is clear that ART to the prostatic bed decreases the serum PSA in cases of persistent disease after RP. What is not clear is why, when the PSA drops 50% or greater in over 80% of patients (and to undetectable levels using routine PSA assays in over 50%), the durability of this suppression is often limited. For example, durable decreases in PSA to undetectable levels lasting longer than a year and a half have been reported in only 25%[43] to 50%[51] of patients.

ART seems to work better when the PSA is very low. For example, decrease in serum PSA to undetectable levels after ART is twice as common in patients who had initially undetectable PSA after RP as those who did not.[30] In fact, the percentage of patients who will drop into the undetectable range after ART is directly related to the level of PSA when they were treated. For example, the percentage of patients who dropped into the undetectable PSA range after ART varies from 29% (PSA 0.6)[52] to 53% (PSA 0.4)[30] to 94% (PSA 0.2).[53]

Less substantial decreases in PSA also occur after ART. Eighty percent of patients with detectable PSA after RP in Abi-Aad's 1992 study showed a PSA decline of 50% or more,[30] while more than 50% of the patients in Hudson's 1990 study had no change in PSA at all after ART.[52] We showed in 1990 that these decreases in PSA are maximal about 6 months after ART is completed.[43] Pathologic grade does not seem to affect the response of PSA,[43] although patients with high Gleason scores and seminal vesicle invasion generally had a less significant drop in PSA after ART.[54]

Some studies have attempted to demonstrate that ART improves cancer relapse rates by comparing their results to published reports of similar patients who did not receive ART. Frazier et al. have asserted that ART in their hands decreases the incidence of biochemically *and* clinically detectable cancer compared to published series where ART is not given.[2] This result was relatively modest when all patients were grouped together (recurrence rate of 51% instead of 64%), however in patients with positive surgical margins, the rate drops more significantly from 64% to 34%. Patients with positive seminal vesicles had a less marked drop from 43% to 36%. As always in prostate cancer research, it is not known if this improved disease-free survival translates into disease specific survival.[23]

In a nonrandomized study at the Mayo Clinic, Cheng et al. supported Frazier's claims by showing that ART improved disease-free survival from 84% to 95%.[18] Disease-specific and crude survival were not affected. Unrandomized comparisons such as this have limited utility, however, because the beneficial effects could be entirely due to patient selection. This difficulty in comparing results of ART to untreated patients in a nonrandomized fashion is demonstrated in a study by Freeman et al.[54] They found that comparing their own 5- and 10-year survival rates of 94% and 70% to those in the literature was difficult, as these rates had a very wide range, from 25% to 92% (5 years) and 6% to 72% (10 years).

Timing of Adjuvant Radiation Therapy

We do not know the best time to give ART. On one hand, early treatment seems like it would be most beneficial, however one would like to avoid treating patients who might not need it. We found no difference in response to treatment when ART was delayed up to 5 years.[43] Zietman et al. found no differences in survival when patients were treated within 3 months or after 6 months of RP.[23]

Dosage of Adjuvant Radiation Therapy

Different total dosages of ART are used in different centers. For example, Massachusetts General Hospital uses 60–64 Gy,[23] while the University of Southern California Hospital uses 45–55 Gy.[54] An approach to dosing has been proposed by Zietman et al.[23] who use 45–55 Gy for those patients with undetectable PSA or specimen-confined T3 disease, and 55–65 Gy for those patients with positive margins. We have chosen at our institution not to exceed 60 Gy, which we feel allows us tumor response with few complications.

Complications of Adjuvant Radiation Therapy

It is generally agreed upon that ART will cause a moderate number of self-limited mild symptoms, but few serious complications. Some researchers noted mild symptoms such as urinary frequency, dysuria, transient hematuria, diarrhea, or proctitis in many of the treated patients.[45,52,54–56] Others feel that these complaints are rare.[30,43,57]

Serious complications do occur in those receiving ART, above what might be expected for RP alone or XRT alone.[58] Specifically, urethral strictures are probably doubled or even trebled from a base rate of 3% after RP to between 6% to 10% after ART.[49,59] Other serious complications such as persistent gross hematuria (5%)[55] and persistent rectal bleeding (5%)[52] have been reported. The grave complication of lower extremity edema after ART is described with a frequency of 3% to 21% in some studies,[45,56,59] but seems have to been eliminated in others.[49,55]

Perhaps one of the greatest concerns for those patients and doctors electing ART is that radiation will cause or worsen incontinence. Despite this fear, most authors have reported no new incontinence after ART.[23,49,54,55,57] Zietman et al. also reported that the time to reach continence was not affected by ART in those patients who received treatment soon after surgery.[23] Isolated cases of incontinence due to ART have been reported, however.[52,58]

Finally, there is no evidence that ART worsens impotence, which is already a significant problem after even nerve sparing RP.[49] Cases of impotence after ART have been reported,[52] but not in such high numbers that ART alone can be implicated.

Detailed analysis of the pre- and post-PSA era literature cannot definitively answer the question of whether or not to give ART. A Southwest Oncology Group (SWOG) study is underway to answer these questions, but the results will not be available for many years. In the meantime, the literature that we have summarized here and elsewhere[60] would suggest the following:

1. ART seems of little benefit if the post-RP PSA does not descend to undetectable levels.
2. ART seems of little value in patients with positive lymph nodes or in those with "significant" seminal vesicle involvement.
3. Patients with initially undetectable post-RP levels that later rise into the detectable range can be placed into two broad categories: those with fast doubling times (< 6 months) who mostly develop systemic disease and those with slow doubling times who usually have only local persistent disease.

Accordingly, we have recently developed an algorithm for deciding on the use of ART[60] (Fig. 5.1). Briefly, if the patient has positive lymph nodes and/or significantly positive seminal vesicles, ART is not advised and hormonal therapy should be considered. If the man has unequivocally positive margins with positive seminal vesicles or lymph nodes, ART may be advisable upon recovery regardless of his postoperative PSA level. If the initial postoperative PSA level is undetectable and the intraoperative and post-RP pathology are equivocal for persistent disease (remembering that 50% of margin positive

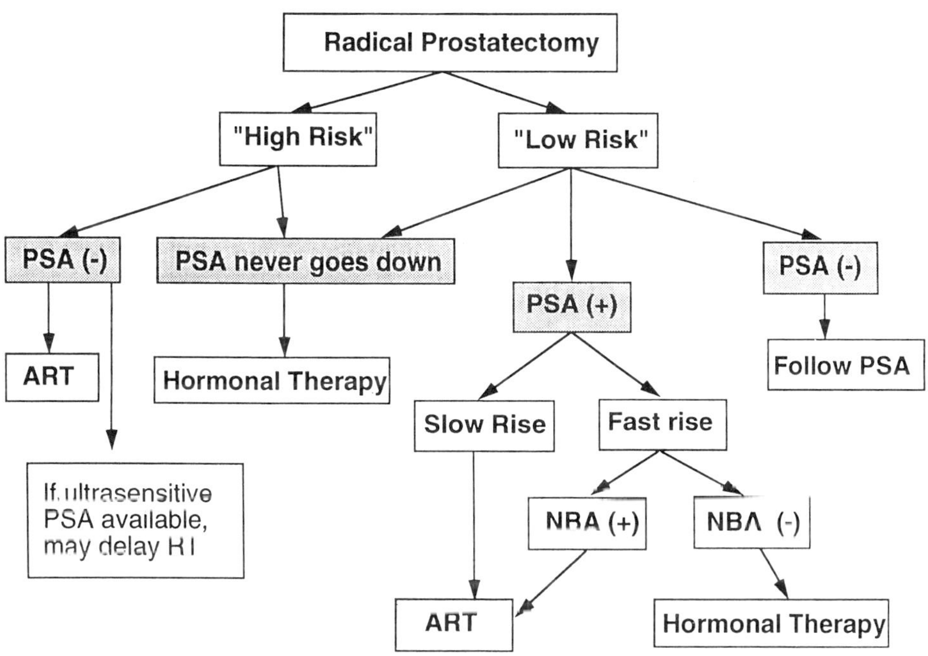

Fig. 5.1. Algorithm for the use of adjuvant radiation therapy. High and low risk are based on pathologic stage and tumor grade. NBA = needle biopsy of the urethrovesical anastomosis. Reprinted from Takayama and Lange, ref. [60], with permission.

disease is cured by RP), ART should be withheld. If the PSA subsequently rises and has a fast doubling time, a biopsy of the prostatic fossa seems prudent: if negative, hormonal therapy should be considered. If this biopsy is positive, ART may be considered, remembering that durable response rates in this group are not high. Finally, if the subsequent PSA rise is slow, ART is advisable in our opinion because this is the group most likely to have a durable response. In this last group, a biopsy of the prostatic fossa is probably not necessary because it could be falsely negative. In all these considerations, the physician should be certain that the PSA is in fact abnormal (a level $>$ 0.1 ng/ml) and is unequivocally elevated over time.

ANTIANDROGEN THERAPY

Although antiandrogen therapy is unquestionably palliative against advanced prostate cancer, there is virtually no information on its effect on persistent disease after RP. What data are available concern the effect of antiandrogens after RP for D1 disease.[54] In this context, local disease but not survival appears to be impacted by the antiandrogen therapy. This mirrors the findings in other studies.[8,52,53] Schellhammer and El-Mahdi felt that salvage antiandrogens after failure of both RP and ART halted growth in one-half of patients.[61] Because antiandrogen therapy is well-tolerated and safe, it can be used to treat persistent disease after RP if the practitioner desires.

There is no question that antiandrogen therapy in patients with persistent cancer after RP lowers the PSA level, and this suppression is often durable. The effects on survival, however, are unknown. A SWOG prospective study comparing antiandrogens to placebo in pathologic C disease is about to begin in order to answer this question.

CYTOTOXIC CHEMOTHERAPY

Determining the efficacy of cytotoxic chemotherapy has been difficult. We know of few studies of the effects of cytotoxics on persistent disease after RP. These have shown an effect of estramustine against local recurrence,[62,63] however, this treatment is risky and carries a nearly 50% risk of serious marrow toxicity. Moreover, 3% of treated patients die rapidly from complications of the therapy.[62]

Other data on the effect of cytotoxic drugs involve their effect against advanced disease and their value here is questionable. However, these studies have shown that advanced prostate cancers can respond to cytotoxic agents,[62] but this has never been shown to improve survival.[64,65] Overall, in the absence of newer data that it helps greatly, cytotoxics should probably be avoided in persistent disease after RP.

REFERENCES

1. Stein A, DeKernion JB, Smith RB, et al: Prostate specific antigen levels after radical prostatectomy in patients with organ confined and locally extensive prostate cancer. *J Urol* 147:942, 1992.
2. Frazier HA, Robertson JE, Humphrey PA, et al: Is prostate specific antigen of clinical importance in evaluating outcome after radical prostatectomy. *J Urol* 149:516, 1993.

3. Jewett HJ: The present status of radical prostatectomy for stages A and B prostatic cancer. *Urol Clin North Am* 2:105, 1975.
4. Schellhammer PF: Radical prostatectomy for carcinoma of the prostate and 15 year analysis of survival and local controls. *J Urol* 135:247A, 1986.
5. Adolfsson J, Steineck G, Whitmore Jr WF: Recent results of management of palbably clinically localized prostate cancer. *Cancer* 72:310, 1993.
6. Anscher MS, Prosnitz LR: Multivariate analysis of factors predicting local relapse after radical prostatectomy—possible indications for postoperative radiotherapy. *Int J Radiat Oncol Biol Phys* 21:941, 1991.
7. Morgan W, Bergstralh EJ, Zincke H: Long-term evaluation of radical prostatectomy as treatment for clinical stage C (T3) prostate cancer. *Urol* 41:113, 1993.
8. Epstein JI, Carmichael M, Partin AW, et al: Is tumor volume an independent predictor of progression following radical prostatectomy: A multivariate analysis of 185 clinical stage B adenocarcinomas of the prostate with 5 years of followup. *J Urol* 149:1478, 1993.
9. Partin AW, Borland RN, Epstein JI, et al: Influence of wide excision of the neurovascular bundles(s) on prognosis in men with clinically localized prostate cancer with established capsular penetration. *J Urol* 150:142, 1993.
10. Oesterling JE, Epstein JI, Walsh PC: Long-term autopsy findings following radical prostatectomy. *Urology* 29:584, 1987.
11. Carter GE, Lieskovsky G, Skinner DG, et al: Results of local and/or systemic adjuvant therapy in the management of pathological stage C or D1 prostate cancer following radical prostatectomy. *J Urol* 142:1266, 1989.
12. Partin AW, Pearson JD, Landis PK, et al: Evaluation of serum prostate-specific antigen velocity after radical prostatectomy to distinguish local recurrence from distant metastases. *Urology* 43:649, 1994.
13. Schellhammer PF: Radical prostatectomy. Patterns of local failure and survival in 67 patients. *Urology* 31:191, 1988.
14. Epstein JI, Carmichael MJ, Pizov G, et al: Influence of capsular penetration on progression following radical prostatectomy: A study of 196 cases with long-term followup. *J Urol* 150:135, 1993.
15. Stamey TA, Kabalin JN, McNeal JE, et al: Prostate specific antigen in the diagnosis and treatment of adenocarcinoma of the prostate. II. Radical prostatectomy treated patients. *J Urol* 141:1076, 1989.
16. Schellhammer PF: Radical prostatectomy: Patterns of local failure and survival in 67 patients. *Urology* 31:191, 1988.
17. McNeal JE, Villers AA, Redwine EA, Freiha FS, Stamey T: Capsular penetration in prostate cancer. Significance for natural history and treatment. *Am J Surg Path* 14:240, 1990.
18. Cheng WS, Frydenberg M, Bergstralh EJ, et al: Radical prostatectomy for pathologic stage C prostate cancer: Influence of pathologic variables and adjuvant treatment on disease outcome. *Urology* 42:282, 1993.
19. Epstein JI: Evaluation of radical prostatectomy capsular margins of resection: The significance of margins designated as negative, closely approaching, and positive. *The Am J Surg Pathol* 14:626, 1990.
20. Paulson DF, Moul JW, Walther PJ: Radical prostatectomy for clinical stage T1-2N0M0 prostatic adenocarcinoma. Long-term results. *J Urol* 144:1180, 1990.
21. Carmichael MJ, Veltri RW, Partin AW, Miller, et al: Deoxyribonucleic acid ploidy analysis as a

predictor of recurrence following radical prostatectomy for stage T2 disease. *J Urol* 153:1015, 1995.

22. Gibbons RP, Cole BS, Richardson RG, et al: Adjuvant radiotherapy following radical prostatectomy: Results and complications. *J Urol* 135:65, 1986.
23. Zietman AL, Coen JJ, Shipley WU, et al: Adjuvant irradiation after radical prostatectomy for adenocarcinoma of prostate: Analysis of freedom from PSA failure. *Urology* 42:292, 1993.
24. Stephenson RA, Middleton RG: Reduction in the rate or positive surgical margins for clinically localized prostate cancer. *J Urol* 151:256A, 1994.
25. McCullough DL, Leadbetter WF: Radical pelvic surgery for locally extensive carcinoma of the prostate. *J Urol* 108:939, 1972.
26. Spaulding JT, Whitmore WF: Extended total excision of prostatic adenocarcinoma. *J Urol* 120:188, 1978.
27. Lightner DJ, Lange PH, Reddy PK, Moore L: Prostate specific antigen and local recurrence after radical prostatectomy. *J Urol* 144:921, 1990.
28. Wasserman NF, Kapoor DA, Hildebrandt WC, Zang G, Born, et al: Transrectal US in evaluation of patients after radical prostatectomy. Part II. Transrectal US and biopsy findings in the presence of residual and early recurrent prostatic cancer. *Radiology* 185:367, 1992.
29. Parra RO, Wolf RM, Huben RP: The use of transrectal ultrasound in the detection and evaluation of local pelvic recurrences after a radical urological pelvic operation. *J Urol* 144:707, 144.
30. Abi-Aad AS, Macfarlane MT, Stein A, et al: Detection of local recurrence after radical prostatectomy by prostate specific antigen and transrectal ultrasound. *J Urol* 147:952, 1992.
31. Takayama TK, Krieger JN, True LD, et al: Recurrent prostate cancer despite undetectable prostate specific antigen. *J Urol* 148:1541, 1992.
32. Kamoshida S, Tsutsumi Y: Extraprostatic localization of prostatic acid phosphatase and prostate-specific antigen: Distribution in cloacogenic glandular epithelium and sex-dependent expression in human anal gland. *Hum Pathol* 21:1108, 1990.
33. Iwakiri J, Grandbois K, Wehner N, Graves HCB, Stamey T: An analysis of urinary prostate specific antigen before and after radical prostatectomy: Evidence for secretion of prostate specific antigen by the periurethral glands. *J Urol* 149:783, 1993.
34. Golz R, Schubert GE: Prostatic specific antigen: Immunoreactivity in urachal remnants. *J Urol* 141:1480, 1989.
35. Oesterling JE, Chan DW, Epstein JI, et al: Prostate specific antigen in the preoperative and postoperative evaluation of localized prostatic cander treated with radical prostatectomy. *J Urol* 139:766, 1988.
36. Lange PH, Ercole CJ, Lightner DJ, et al: The value of serum prostate specific antigen determinations before and after radical prostatectomy. *J Urol* 141:873, 1989.
37. Danella J, Steckel J, Dorey F, et al: Detectable prostate specific antigen levels following radical prostatectomy: Relationship of doubling time to clinical outcome. *J Urol* 149:447A, 1993.
38. Takayama TK, Vessella RL, Brawer MK, et al: The enhanced detection of persistent disease after prostatectomy with a new prostate specific antigen immunoassay. *J Urol* 150:374, 1993.
39. Shinohara K, Presti JCJ, Ingerman A, et al: Local recurrence after radical prostatectomy: characteristics in size, location and PSA. *J Urol* 151:256A, 1994.
40. Foster LS, Jajodia P, Fournier GJ, et al: The value of prostate specific antigen and transrectal ultrasound guided biopsy in detecting prostatic fossa recurrences following radical prostatectomy. *J Urol* 149:1024, 1993.
41. Stamey TA, Graves HCB, Wehner N, et al: Early detection of residual prostate cancer after rad-

ical prostatectomy by an ultrasensitive assay for prostate specific antigen. *J Urol* 149:787, 1993.

42. Wasserman NF, Kapoor DA, Hildebrandt WC, et al: Transrectal US in evaluation of patients after radical prostatectomy. Part I. Normal postoperative anatomy. *Radiology* 185:361, 1992.
43. Lange PH, Lightner DJ, Medini E, et al: The effect of radiation therapy after radical prostatectomy in patients with elevated prostate specific antigen levels. *J Urol* 144:927, 1990.
44. Fowler Jr JE, Brooks J, Pandey P, et al: Variable histology of anastamotic biopsies with detectable prostate specific antigen after radical prostatectomy. *J Urol* 153:1011, 1995.
45. Jacobson GM, Smith JAJ, Stewart JR: Postoperative radiation therapy for pathologic stage C prostate cancer. *Int J Radiat Oncol Biol Phys* 13:1021, 1987.
46. Rosen EM, Cassady JR, Connolly J, et al: Radiotherapy for localized prostate cancer. *Int J Radiat Oncol Biol Phys* 10:2201, 1984.
47. Kabalin JN, Hodge KK, McNeal JE, et al: Identification of residual cancer in the prostate following radiation therapy: Role of transrectal ultrasound guided biopsy and prostate specific antigen. *J Urol* 142:326, 1989.
48. Paulson DF, Moul JW, Robertson JE, et al: Postoperative radiotherapy of the prostate for patients undergoing radical prostatectomy with positive margins, seminal vesicle involvement and/or penetration through the capsule. *J Urol* 143:1178, 1990.
49. Meier R, Mark R, St. Royal, et al: Postoperative radiation therapy after radical prostatectomy for prostate carcinoma. *Cancer* 70:1960, 1992.
50. Shevlin BE, Mittal BB, Brand WN, et al: The role of adjuvant irradiation following primary prostatectomy, based on histopathologic extent of tumor. *Int J Radiat Oncol Biol Phys* 16:1425, 1989.
51. Link P, Freiha FS, Stamey TA: Adjuvant radiation therapy in patients with detectable prostate specific antigen following radical prostatectomy. *J Urol* 145:532, 1991.
52. Hudson M, Catalona WJ: Effect of adjuvant radiation therapy on prostate specific antigen following radical prostatectomy. *J Urol* 143:1174, 1990.
53. Morgan WR, Zincke H, Rainwater LM, et al: Prostate specific antigen values after radical retropubic prostatectomy for adenocarcinoma of the prostate: Impact of adjuvant treatment (hormonal and radiation). *J Urol* 145:319, 1991.
54. Freeman JA, Lieskovsky G, Cook DW, et al: Radical retropubic prostatectomy and postoperative radiation for pathological stage C (PCN0) Prostate cancer from 1976 to 1989: Intermediate findings. *J Urol* 149:1029, 1993.
55. Hanks GE, Dawson AK: The role of external beam radiation therapy after prostatectomy for prostate cancer. *Cancer* 58:2406, 1986.
56. Petrovich Z, Lieskovsky G, Langholz B, et al: Radiotherapy following radical prostatectomy in patients with adenocarcinoma of the prostate. *Int J Radiat Oncol Biol Phys* 21:949, 1991.
57. Pilepich MV, Walz BJ, Baglan RJ: Postoperative irradiation in carcinoma of the prostate. *Int J Radiat Oncol Biol Phys* 10:1869, 1984.
58. Ray GR, Bagshaw MA, Freiha F: External beam radiation salvage for residual or recurrent local tumor following radical prostatectomy. *J Urol* 132:926, 1984.
59. Forman JD, Wharam MD, Lee DJ, et al: Definitive radiotherapy following prostatectomy: Results and complications. *Int J Radiat Oncol Biol Phys* 12:185, 1986.
60. Takayama TK, Lange PH: Radiation therapy for local recurrence of prostate cancer after radical prostatectomy. *Urol Clin North Am* 21:687, 1994.
61. Schellhammer PF, El-Mahdi AM: Local failure and relative complications after definitive treat-

ment of carcinoma of the prostate by irradiation or surgery. *Urol Clin North Am* 17:835, 1990.

62. Schmidt JD: Cytotoxic agents effective in prostate cancer. *Semin Urol* 1:299, 1983.
63. Schmidt JD, Gibbons RP, Murphy GP, et al: Adjuvant therapy for localized prostate cancer. *Cancer* 71:1005, 1993.
64. Eisenberger MA, Bezerdkian L, Kalash S: A critical assessment of the role of chemotherapy for endocrine-resistant prostatic carcinoma. *Urol Clin North Am* 14:695, 1987.
65. Yagoda A: Cytotoxic agents in prostate cancer: an enigma. *Semin Urol* 1:311, 1983.

6

The Current Role of Radical Perineal Prostatectomy in Localized Prostatic Cancer

Richard G. Middleton

Seventy years ago in *Young's Practice of Urology*, Hugh Young described very well the perineal exposure of the prostate for perineal simple prostatic enucleation and for radical perineal prostatectomy in the case of a localized prostate cancer.[1] Young's description of the technique of perineal exposure has not been surpassed, and his writing was liberally illustrated by William Didusch's superb anatomic drawings. Young's section on perineal surgery is still worth the attention of urologists and urologic residents who want a detailed guide to a virtually bloodless and anatomic procedure for exposing and removing the prostate. For many decades since the era of Hugh Young, a number of urologic surgeons have reported their generally favorable experience with radical perineal prostatectomy in well selected cases of clinically localized prostatic cancer.

Notable proponents of radical perineal prostatectomy have been Jewett,[2] Belt,[3] Culp,[4] Hodges,[5] Gibbons,[6] and Goodwin.[7] Elmer Belt, a urologist who had a huge experience with perineal surgery, modified Young's surgical technique by a method of entering the perineum underneath the anal sphincter mechanism.[8] To this day some perineal surgeons use Young's inverted U-shaped perineal incision coming directly into the perineum over, or anterior to, the sphincter muscles; while others use the Belt approach with a flatter transverse incision, staying close to the rectal wall and developing a plane to the prostate underneath the sphincter muscles—between the anal sphincter and the anterior rectal wall.

Many urologic surgeons have called attention to some of the appealing aspects of the perineal approach to radical prostatectomy. The operation can usually be accomplished relatively quickly with low blood loss. The patient has minimal postoperative pain and no postoperative ileus, so he can begin oral fluid and food intake immediately after surgery. The deep dorsal veins, a significant concern during radical retropubic prostatectomy, are generally avoided during perineal prostatectomy. Also the anastomosis of the bladder neck to membranous urethra can be performed precisely under direct vision via the perineal route.

With the current focus upon reducing the time of a patient's postoperative hospital stay, radical perineal prostatectomy should be very popular. Discharge on the second or third postoperative day is quite reasonable. Also postoperative convalescence is easier and return to normal physical energy and stamina is quicker than for the patient recovering from a lower abdominal incision.

While there are distinct advantages to the radical perineal operation over the radical retropubic prostatectomy, some concerns about the perineal prostatectomy should be noted: (1) Perineal prostatectomy requires considerable experience and a good teacher. (2) Rectal injury is more common until the surgeon gains considerable experience. (3) Staging pelvic lymphadenectomy either requires a separate operative procedure or is omitted. (4) Concerns have been expressed that an "extended" radical prostatectomy and a nerve-sparing prostatectomy may be more difficult to accomplish perineally compared to retropubic surgery.

Historically radical perineal prostatectomy has been underutilized. Radical perineal prostatectomy for localized prostate cancer has never gained wide popularity among urologists. There have been three reasons, this author believes, why the procedure has not been commonly employed, and why urologists for many decades were content to send their patients for radiation therapy rather than pursue a surgical solution for localized prostate cancer. Learning radical perineal prostatectomy requires time, experience, and an enthusiastic teacher. Too few urologic training programs have had the experienced teachers necessary to instruct residents in perineal techniques. The inexperienced perineal surgeon has usually had great fear of causing a rectal injury. Furthermore, staging of the cancer was inaccurate and primitive during the era when perineal prostatectomy was the only recognized surgical procedure for early or localized cancer.

THE RISE OF RADICAL RETROPUBIC PROSTATECTOMY

During the past 15 years there has been a phenomenal rise in the use of radical retropubic prostatectomy for localized prostate cancer. The operation is now undertaken by the majority of urologists in the United States and is taught to residents in all urologic training programs. With the great rise in interest in surgical treatment, urologists have lost their previous enthusiasm for external beam radiation as primary treatment for localized prostate cancer.

Some of the reasons for the popularity of radical retropubic prostatectomy among urologists today are: (1) Today's urologist is comfortable, experienced, and trained to operate in the pelvis. (2) Lymphadenectomy for staging can be carried out at the same time and through the same incision used for removal of the prostate. (3) New technology, specifically, prostate specific antigen (PSA), prostatic ultrasound, and ultrasound-directed prostate biopsies have helped identify many more patients who have truly early and localized prostate cancer and are likely to benefit from radical prostatectomy. (4) The use of post-treatment PSA and post-treatment biopsy have shown external beam radiation therapy to have a lower curative rate than was previously thought. Urologists have become disenchanted with external beam radiation therapy as their enthusiasm has increased for radical retropubic prostatectomy. (5) The development of a nerve-sparing or potency-sparing radical prostatectomy has increased the interest in surgical therapy of localized prostate cancer.

TWO-STAGE RADICAL PROSTATECTOMY

During the 1970s and early 1980s our common approach to clinically localized prostate cancer at the University of Utah was a two-stage operation. The first stage was a pelvic lymphadenectomy. This was performed through a low midline abdominal incision, or by sequential lower abdominal muscle splitting extraperitoneal procedures. Since this was a staging procedure, the second or contralateral pelvic node dissection was omitted when positive, or tumor-bearing nodes, were discovered on the first side. When nodes were normal, or seemed normal, the contralateral lymph node dissection was performed. If permanent histologic sections showed no nodal metastases, radical perineal prostatectomy was carried out—usually 3 or 4 days after the pelvic lymphadenectomy and usually during the same hospital admission. When permanent sections indicated positive pelvic nodes, no second stage or radical prostatectomy was performed. During this era, we reported our experience with pelvic lymphadenectomy in 452 patients.[9] No patient with stage A1 prostate cancer had nodal metastases, while 24% of patients with stage A2 cancer had positive nodes. The incidence of pelvic nodal metastasis was 12% in clinical stage B1 tumors and 28% in clinical stage B2 prostate cancer. Also, tumor grade influenced the incidence of tumor-bearing pelvic nodes within each stage. It became clear that pelvic lymphadenectomy was unnecessary in stage A1 tumors (and radical prostatectomy also seemed unnecessary). Patients with low-grade (Gleason score 2, 3, 4) cancers that were clinically stage B1 had only a 4% incidence of positive nodes—such a low incidence that lymphadenectomy for staging was later omitted. A decision whether or not to proceed with radical prostatectomy seemed to require histologic examination of the nodes in stage A2, medium- and high-grade B1 tumors and all B2 lesions.

Delay of a radical prostatectomy for several days, until permanent histologic sections of the lymph nodes were analyzed, resulted in no false-negative node results. On the other hand, the delay between the two stages while waiting for the result of the lymphadenectomy was frustrating for the patient and for the surgeon. Nonetheless, this was a reasonable and effective method for dealing with clinically localized prostate cancer.

LAPAROSCOPIC PELVIC LYMPHADENECTOMY PLUS RADICAL PERINEAL PROSTATECTOMY

Many urologists in recent years have reported their experience with laparoscopic removal of pelvic lymph nodes as an alternative to open surgical lymph node dissection. Pelvic lymph nodes can be removed transperitoneally or through an extraperitoneal laparoscopic approach. Laparoscopic lymphadenectomy requires special training and experience, but it can be an effective method to investigate the status of the pelvic lymph nodes in a minimally invasive way. Thus the discovery of positive nodes can allow the patient to avoid an open surgical procedure which is unlikely to be helpful to him. Also, the discovery of normal lymph nodes can allow for radical perineal prostatectomy which is less of an ordeal for the patient than the retropubic radical prostatectomy. Thomas et al. reported a favorable experience with combined laparoscopic pelvic lymphadenectomy and radical perineal prostatectomy when frozen section examination of the pelvic nodes was negative.[10] Advantages included early hospital discharge, low morbidity, and rapid return to normal physical activity. Parra, Lerner, Levy and Resnick, and Wolfe et al. have reported similar experiences with low blood loss, quicker hospital discharge, and fewer complications when radical perineal prostatectomy replaced radical retropubic prostatectomy.[11–14]

RADICAL PERINEAL PROSTATECTOMY WITHOUT PELVIC LYMPHADENECTOMY

Twelve years ago, in analyzing our data from pelvic lymphadenectomy and radical prostatectomy, we discovered that our patients who were clinical stage A2 with well-differentiated prostate cancer (Gleason score 2, 3, and 4) had a 0% incidence of positive pelvic lymph nodes. Of patients with well-differentiated clinical B1 cancers, (Gleason score 2,3, 4) only 4% had positive pelvic lymph nodes. It seemed reasonable, therefore, to omit pelvic lymphadenectomy in those patients with low-grade stage A2 and B1 lesions; the likelihood of nodal metastasis was insignificant.

Recently several authors have pointed out that a PSA level of less than 10 ng/ml also indicates a low likelihood of pelvic nodal metastasis. Patients with only grade 2 and 3 prostatic adenocarcinoma and a PSA of under 10.0 have such a low level of positive pelvic lymph nodes that a staging lymphadenectomy seems unnecessary. Incidentally, these same patients also do not need preoperative bone scans—bone metastasis in this context is extremely rare.

Certainly radical perineal prostatectomy is an appealing choice for the patient with a low-grade tumor and a PSA under 10.0.

The patient whose tumor contains grade 4 or 5 elements or has a PSA greater than 10 ng/ml (or both) has a significant risk of metastasis to pelvic nodes and may not benefit significantly from radical prostatectomy; so omission of node dissection in these patients is not reasonable. Radical perineal prostatectomy is an appropriate procedure, but only when the nodes have been proven normal.

ARE THERE DISADVANTAGES TO THE RADICAL PERINEAL PROSTATECTOMY?

Patient Positioning

Perineal prostatectomy requires placing the patient in an exaggerated perineal position. This may be impossible in the patient with limited mobility of his hips. Extreme obesity can also make positioning difficult and interfere with adequate exposure of the prostate. Positioning is very important for prostate exposure, but it is extremely important to have adequate padding for the legs and to avoid knee pressure on the patient's chest. Rhabdomyolysis and acute renal failure have been reported from prolonged pressure against leg muscles during perineal prostatectomy.[15] It should be noted that radical perineal prostatectomy can be carried out very effectively in the patient who has already had an abdominoperineal resection of his rectum.

Incontinence

Some authors have reported higher rates of postoperative urinary incontinence after radical perineal prostatectomy, whereas others have stated that continence rates are better after radical perineal prostatectomy compared to radical retropubic prostatectomy. Advocates of perineal prostatectomy point to better visualization in performing an accurate anastomosis of the bladder neck to membranous urethra. At the University of Utah we compared postoperative continence in 70 patients who had radical retropubic prostatectomy with 70 patients who underwent radical perineal prostatectomy.[16] The results were equal in the percentages with early good control and time to achieve good control in those with postoperative stress incontinence.

Impotence

Thanks to Walsh, urologists understand the techniques necessary to carry out a nerve-sparing or potency-sparing radical retropubic prostatectomy. Modifications have been suggested and reported to accomplish the same nerve sparing goal through a perineal route. Certainly potency has been preserved during the perineal procedure, but further data are needed to understand the incidence of preserved potency after perineal prostatectomy.

The Extended Radical Prostatectomy

A technique has been described in Chapter 4 for widening the margins of the radical prostatectomy specimen by encompassing more of the periprostatic tissue. This method had been developed for radical retropubic prostatectomy, but the authors do not believe that the same extended margins can be as effectively developed via the perineal route. Further study of this problem is underway.

Rectal Injury

Injury, or entrance into the rectum, has been common in perineal exposure of the prostate. Clearly, fear of rectal injury has discouraged many urologists from developing their skills in perineal prostatectomy. Experience, patience, and good instruction are needed before a surgeon can expose the prostate and preserve the rectal integrity with confidence. Good preoperative bowel preparation is important. Most injuries can be repaired carefully in the presence of a clean rectum, with a low likelihood of ultimate rectourinary fistula.

A reliable and safe method for repair of rectourinary fistula, should it occur, is important for the surgeon's confidence and the patient's well-being. The author strongly recommends the posterior York-Mason procedure; this is described in detail in Chapter 7.

SUMMARY

Radical perineal prostatectomy has never been widely popular or widely employed by American urologic surgeons. There have been strong advocates of the perineal operation who have persevered in gaining experience and confidence with the procedure. The results for the proponents of this procedure have been a quicker, highly effective radical prostatectomy with low blood loss, less operative pain, and an easier recovery for the patient.

Pelvic lymph node assessment by laparoscopy and the recognition that selected patients with low-grade tumors and a low PSA do not need lymphadenectomy at all make perineal prostatectomy an appealing alternative at times.

Fear of rectal injury has been an obstacle, but proper technique and preparation of the patient can greatly reduce this problem. And a reliable technique for the repair of rectourinary fistula is available.

Enthusiasm for the procedure is justified, and better training in perineal surgery for urologists and urologic residents is recommended.

REFERENCES

1. Young HH, Davis DM: *Young's Practice of Urology, Vol II. Operations on the Prostate.* Philadelphia, WB Saunders, 1926, p 414.
2. Jewett HJ: The case for radical perineal prostatectomy. *J Urol* 103:195, 1970.
3. Belt E, Schroeder FH: Total perineal prostatectomy for carcinoma of the prostate. *J Urol* 107:91, 1972.
4. Culp OS, Meyer JJ: Radical prostatectomy in the treatment of prostatic cancer. *Cancer* 32:1113, 1973.
5. Hodges CV, Pearse HD, Stille L: Radical prostatectomy for carcinoma: 30-year experience and 15-year survivals. *J Urol* 122:180, 1979.
6. Gibbons RP, Correa RJ Jr, Brannan GE, et al: Total prostatectomy for localized prostatic cancer. *J Urol* 131:73, 1984.
7. Boxer RJ, Kaufman JJ, Goodwin WE: Radical prostatectomy for carcinoma of the prostate: 1951–1976. A review of 329 patients. *J Urol* 117:208, 1977.
8. Belt E, Ebert CE, Surber AC Jr: A new anatomic approach in perineal prostatectomy. *J Urol* 41:482, 1939.
9. Smith JA Jr, Seaman JP, Gleidman JB, et al: Pelvic lymph node metastasis from prostatic cancer: influence of tumor grade and stage in 452 consecutive patients. *J Urol* 130:290, 1983.
10. Thomas R, Steele R, Smith R, et al: One-stage laparoscopic pelvic lymphadenectomy and radical perineal prostatectomy. *J Urol* 152:1174, 1994.
11. Parra RO, Boullier JA, Rauscher JA, et al: The value of laparoscopic lymphadenectomy in conjunction with radical perineal or retropubic prostatectomy. *J Urol* 151:1599, 1994.
12. Lerner SE, Fleischman J, Taub HC, et al: Combined laparoscopic pelvic lymph node dissection and modified Belt radical perineal prostatectomy for localized prostatic adenocarcinoma. *Urology* 43:493, 1994.
13. Levy DA, Resnick MI: Laparoscopic pelvic lymphadenectomy and radical perineal prostatectomy: a viable alternative to radical retropubic prostatectomy. *J Urol* 151:905, 1994.

14. Wolfe JS Jr, Shinohara K, Kerlikowske KM, et al: Selection of patients for laparoscopic pelvic lymphadenectomy prior to radical prostatectomy: a decision analysis. *Urology* 42:680, 1993.

15. Ali H, Nieto JG, Rhamy RK, et al: Acute renal failure due to rhabdomyolysis associated with the extreme lithotomy position. *Am J Kidney Dis* 22:865, 1993.

16. Unpublished data.

7

The Management of Rectal Injury Associated with Radical Prostatectomy

Richard G. Middleton
Robert A. Stephenson

RECTAL INJURY DURING RADICAL PROSTATECTOMY

Rectal injury, or inadvertent entry into the rectum, has been reported to occur in 0 to 5.4% of cases of radical prostatectomy. Most reports give an incidence of 1–3%. From the University of Utah we reported five rectal injuries in 153 radical prostatectomies (both retropubic and perineal) performed from 1970 to 1980.[1] In four of five cases, immediate repair of the rectum without colostomy was successful. One immediate repair was not successful, and a rectourinary fistula developed. From a very large experience with radical retropubic prostatectomy at the Mayo Clinic, Zincke et al. reported a 1.5% incidence of rectal injury before 1988, with a reduced rate of 0.6% since 1988.[2]

Because of the well-recognized possibility of rectal entry, the patient undergoing radical prostatectomy should at least have a thorough mechanical bowel preparation prior to surgery. The use of antibiotics preoperatively is optional. When rectal injury is recognized and a careful two-layer surgical repair is accomplished in the presence of a clean rectum, little harm is likely to result from this event. Another measure which has been advocated by some surgeons is the mobilization of omentum from within the peritoneal cavity to interpose between the rectal repair and the bladder neck to membranous urethral anastomosis. Omental mobilization is usually possible during radical retropubic prostatectomy, but it may be very difficult or impossible from the perineal route.

A colostomy can usually be avoided. A colostomy should be considered, however, when the rectal injury is extensive, when closure of the laceration is difficult or considered technically unsatisfactory, when there is a spill of fecal material because of inadequate preoperative bowel preparation, or when there has been previous radiation, as in a "salvage" radical prostatectomy.

The failure of the urologic surgeon to recognize the rectal injury is a serious matter; every effort by the surgeon should be made to inspect the rectum repeatedly during the performance of radical retropubic prostatectomy—and especially a final inspection should be made just prior to the placement of sutures for the bladder neck to membranous urethral anastomosis. The failure to recognize the injury will result in extravasation of infected fecal matter with a local abscess and very likely a communication with the anterior anastomotic region to form a rectourinary fistula. The patient will ultimately drain fecal material from the urethral catheter or urine from the rectum, or both.

Rectal injury during perineal exposure for radical perineal prostatectomy is a significant risk until the surgeon gains proficiency and becomes an expert at mobilization of the rectum from the apical region of the prostate. Once the apex has been precisely mobilized, further risk of rectal injury is diminished greatly. Here again, preoperative bowel preparation is mandatory. When rectal injury occurs with radical perineal prostatectomy, it is usually early in the procedure before the prostate is mobilized and removed; so the surgeon has the option to close the laceration and postpone the radical prostatectomy until another day. When the injury can be repaired well in the presence of a clean rectum, it is permissible to proceed with the radical perineal prostatectomy with a low likelihood of further trouble.

When the rectal injury has been carefully repaired, and colostomy seems unnecessary, a further safeguard is vigorous dilatation of the anal sphincter. This maneuver will reduce the sphincter tone for a time and decreases the likelihood of rectal gas under pressure penetrating the site of repair.

RECTOURINARY FISTULA

Rectourinary fistula is an uncommon problem, but the urologic surgeon will encounter this complication on occasion. Over a 25-year period at the University of Utah we have operated upon 17 patients with rectourinary fistulas. Our early experience has been reported previously.[3-5] Of the 17 with rectourinary fistula, eight patients developed a fistula following radical retropubic prostatectomy; two fistulas occurred after radical perineal prostatectomy; four fistulas resulted from transurethral resection of the prostate; and in one case each a fistula followed simple retropubic prostatectomy, bladder neck reconstruction, and pelvic trauma. Nearly half, or 8 of 17 of our cases of rectourinary fistula occurred after radical retropubic prostatectomy. In most instances the radical prostatectomy was not performed at our institution, but the patient was referred for surgical treatment when the fistula became evident. Nearly always the surgeon had been unaware of the presence of a rectal injury at the time of the radical prostatectomy. It certainly seems that a rectal entry that is unrecognized is far more likely to lead to a rectourinary fistula than an injury that is recognized and properly repaired.

A rectourinary fistula is dramatic. Either the patient passes obvious fecal matter in his urine (usually through the Foley catheter), or urine drains from the rectum. Commonly both types of abnormal drainage occur. There may or may not be fever. The fistula can usually be palpated on rectal examination in the anterior rectal wall. The fistula is usually visualized cystoscopically and can be documented by cystourethrography or barium enema. Our preferred approach for repair of the fistula is the York-Mason posterior transsphincteric, transrectal operation which will be described in detail. First, though, other procedures in the urologic literature for dealing with a rectourinary fistula are reviewed with comments.

Colostomy Plus Indwelling Urethral Catheter or Suprapubic Cystostomy

It is traditional and safe, conservative surgical practice to perform a diverting colostomy at once when a rectourinary fistula is recognized. Urine passing through the fistula can be greatly diminished with bladder drainage—either a suprapubic cystotomy or Foley urethral catheter. Small fistulas will sometimes heal with diversion alone, but time for healing is uncertain. Also, spontaneous healing may not occur at all. The waiting and the uncertainty of outcome are often demoralizing to the patient and the surgeon.

Repair of the Fistula Site Through a Dilated but Intact Anal Sphincter

Through this route the fistula can be excised and repaired in layers.[6] While this method can be successful, better exposure is accomplished by the York-Mason operation.

Perineal Exposure with Excision and Repair of the Fistula

The perineal approach has been described by several authors.[7,8] It is a reasonable approach to rectourinary fistula, but it is a more difficult operation generally than the York-Mason procedure. Preliminary colostomy has often, but not always, been employed.

Transvesical Approach to the Fistula

This method should be avoided because exposure is usually inadequate and there is little room to deal with the fistula in the edematous tissue of the bladder neck and trigone.

Abdominoperineal Mobilization of the Rectosigmoid Colon, Division of the Rectum from the Anal Sphincter, and Pull-through

The rectosigmoid colon is moved caudally to bring healthy colon up against the urinary fistula. Excessive distal colon including the damaged segment is excised. The dissection of the rectosigmoid to permit this mobilization and pull-through can be a formidable and difficult operation. Also fecal control has been compromised by this procedure. The major complaint with this operation is that it can be long and difficult with significant morbidity and a long time for recovery. There are simpler and more effective methods for dealing with the fistula.

THE YORK-MASON APPROACH TO RECTOURINARY FISTULA

Sixteen of our 17 cases of rectourinary fistula have occurred following urologic surgery (most commonly radical prostatectomy), and in one case, the fistula followed perineal trauma. None of our patients had previous radiation therapy. The first nine patients in our series had a preliminary colostomy prior to the York-Mason fistula repair. In recent years we have not performed a preliminary colostomy but have gone ahead with the procedure directly after the patient has a vigorous and thorough mechanical and antibiotic bowel preparation. Our experience has taught us that the preliminary colostomy is usually not necessary.

The patient receives a general anesthetic and is placed in a prone, jackknife position. Tape is used to spread the buttocks. After suitable skin preparation and draping, an incision is made from the posterior anal verge cephalad through the anal sphincter, and this incision is continued up through the posterior wall of the rectum to the tip of the coccyx[9,10] (Fig. 7.1). If the surgeon wants additional length it is possible to amputate the coccyx and extend the incision further cephalad. Also, as an alternative, the surgeon can deviate the incision to the side and extend it up along the lateral border of the coccyx and the distal sacrum. As one cuts across the anal sphincter mechanism, stitches are placed on each side of the divided bundles and tagged with matching clamps so that these bundles can be reapproximated later.

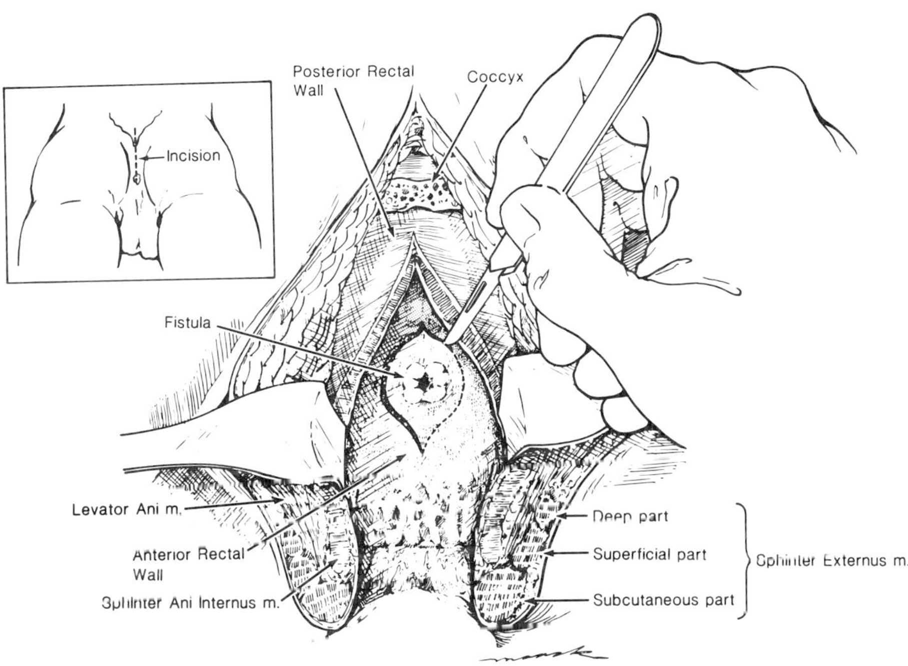

Fig. 7.1. Posterior trans-anal and transrectal exposure of rectourinary fistula.

Lateral retractors are employed inside the rectum, and the surgeon is provided with an excellent direct view of the rectal side of the fistula. An oval or elliptical excision of the entire fistula tract can be accomplished under excellent vision. This excision includes the fistula in the wall of the rectum and its junction with the bladder neck or proximal urethra deeply. With a urethral catheter in place, the edges of the bladder neck or urethra can be sutured with interrupted chromic 2-0 catgut sutures. Next the anterior rectal wall is mobilized on both sides; this allows for a good second layer of closure of anterior rectal muscle with interrupted chromic 2-0 catgut sutures. Finally the third layer is a closure of the mucosa, and usually this is accomplished with a running chromic catgut suture. Three layers of closure are regularly obtained.

After closure of the site of the fistula in three layers, the posterior rectum and anal sphincter are reconstituted. The posterior rectal wall is closed with a continuous suture of 2-0 chromic catgut reinforced with interrupted sutures of the same material. The individual bundles of the anal sphincter are brought together to reapproximate the anus. A small Penrose drain is placed alongside the posterior rectal wall, and the subcutaneous fat and skin are closed superficially.

In years past, we attempted to postpone bowel activity by the placing the patient on intravenous fluids, nothing by mouth (NPO) and narcotic drugs as a constipating regimen. We no longer believe these measures are necessary, and now patients are given a general diet with stool softeners: no effort is made to postpone bowel activity.

Results of the York-Mason Operation for Rectourinary Fistula

In 16 or 17 cases fistula repair was totally successful without fistula recurrence. In one case the fistula persisted or recurred, probably because of inadequate excision of the fistula tract. Three months later a repeat operation with wider excision of the fistula tract was accomplished, and the fistula has remained closed following that operation. Thus the procedure has been a total success in 16 cases, and in one case a repeat operation was necessary, but the result here too was successful.

The operation is performed relatively quickly, in 1 or 2 hr, and it is accomplished with remarkably good exposure. There have been no complications, and specifically there has not been one incident of anal stricture or anal incontinence. Blood loss has been minimal, and no blood transfusions have been given. The York-Mason procedure is recommended as an efficient and highly successful method for closure of rectourinary fistulas. Rectourinary fistula has often been regarded by surgeons as a difficult and formidable complication, but success with this procedure has caused us to lose our fear of this problem.

Rectourinary fistula can be avoided by close inspection of the rectum during radical prostatectomy—or during any urologic procedure performed close to the rectum. Rectal injury occurs occasionally, but when properly repaired a fistula is a rare event. It is the unrecognized rectal injury which most often leads to rectourinary fistula.

REFERENCES

1. Middleton RG, Smith JA Jr, Melzer RB, et al: Patient survival and local recurrence rate following radical prostatectomy for prostatic carcinoma. *J Urol* 136:422, 1986.

2. Zincke H, Oesterling JE, Blute ML, et al: Long-term (15 years) results after radical prostatectomy for clinically localized (Stage T2c or lower) prostate cancer. *J Urol* 152:1850, 1994.
3. Dahl DS, Howard PM, Middleton RG: The surgical management of rectourinary fistulas resulting from a prostatic operation: a report of 5 cases. *J Urol* 111:514, 1974.
4. Henderson DJ, Middleton RG, Dahl DS: Single stage repair of rectourinary fistula. *J Urol* 125:592, 1981.
5. Wood TW, Middleton RG: Single-stage transrectal transsphincteric (modified York-Mason) repair of rectourinary fistulas. *Urology* 35:27, 1990.
6. Vose SN: A technique for the repair of recto-urethral fistula. *J Urol* 61:790, 1949.
7. Culp OS, Calhoon HW: A variety of rectourethral fistulas: experiences with 20 cases. *J Urol* 91:560, 1964.
8. Goodwin WE, Turner RD, Winter CC: Rectourinary fistula: principles of management and a technique of surgical closure. *J Urol* 80:246, 1958.
9. Kilpatrick FR, York-Mason A: Post-operative recto-prostatic fistula. *Br J Urol* 41:649, 1969.
10. Beneventi FA, Cassebaum WH: Rectal flap repair of prostatorectal fistula. *Surg Gynecol Obstet* 133:489, 1971.

8

Management of Node-Positive Prostate Cancer

James E. Montie

In a disease characterized by controversy in many areas, the uncertainty evident in the ideal management of node-positive prostate cancer (PCa) is particularly disconcerting. In addition to the inherent difficulties in studying PCa, the common clinical paradigms of the disease are evolving rapidly; detection (and thus extent of disease at diagnosis) has improved dramatically utilizing prostate specific antigen (PSA). One is confronted with a "Catch-22" situation: meaningful data on PCa outcomes are only evident after 5–10 years of follow-up but the common patient of 5–10 years ago may not be representative of the common case seen now. With a moving target, it is difficult to arrive at firm recommendations. Nevertheless, in the following chapter several facets of the dilemma surrounding the management of node-positive PCa will be reviewed in an effort to provide some guidance for the clinician.

HISTORICAL CONTEXT

In most solid, epithelial cancers, spread into regional lymph nodes vastly worsens the prognosis. Historically, the presence of lymph node metastases from PCa altered the prognosis so much that the finding of positive nodes was equivalent to incurability; up to 75% of men with positive nodes would be expected to develop bone metastases in 5 years.[1] Because the outlook was so dismal, lymph node metastases were felt to preclude attempts at curative local treatment that may itself have inherent morbidity. A lymph node metastasis in essence was equivalent to systemic disease; thus a radical prostatectomy (RP) or definitive radiation therapy (RT) were ill-advised and therapeutically overaggressive. Why subject the patient to the risk of incontinence, impotence, or radiation proctitis if the treatment was destined to fail because of systemic disease? The impact on outcome of positive lymph nodes was so profound that a staging pelvic lymph node dissection (PLND) became an integral part of therapy decisions.[2,3]

PLND became widely accepted in the 1970s. In one of the largest surgical series of PLND prior to RP, Smith et al. found positive lymph nodes in 23% of 452 men with clinically localized PCa.[1] Using the predominant philosophy evident at that time, the RP was abandoned if any lymphatic spread was found; close observation with later RT or endocrine therapy was advised. Similar observations were noted prior to RT with a higher frequency of nodal metastases, presumably because of bulkier local disease. In 300 PLND cases prior to iodine-125 implant, Fowler and Whitmore found a 40% incidence of positive nodes.[3] Performing a more extensive pelvic dissection including hypogastric lymph nodes, McDowell et al. found a 57% incidence of nodal metastases in men with clinical T1–T3 disease.[2] Thus, positive lymph nodes were not only an important prognostic factor but also were identified in a substantial proportion of men.

Later in the 1980s, the clinical circumstances surrounding the detection of PCa began to change. The first important change was brought on by transrectal ultrasound guided biopsy, especially with the availability of a spring-loaded biopsy instrument; this transformed biopsy of the prostate from a procedure requiring general anesthesia to a relatively painless one done in the office. Thus, subtle abnormalities on digital rectal examination were pursued with a biopsy rather than later re-exam. Later in the decade, PSA gradually became more commonly used in the detection of PCa, further shifting the stage at diagnosis to smaller lesions more likely to be confined within the prostate.[4] Concurrent with this apparent earlier detection, a consistent decrease in the frequency of involved lymph nodes was noted. Petros and Catalona found only 6.7% of 518 men had nodal metastases with a PLND prior to RP.[5] Similarly, Danella et al. identified positive nodes in 5.7% of 232 men operated on from 1989 through 1991.[6] Although referral patterns to larger academic centers noted for nerve-sparing surgical techniques might contribute to the preponderance of early cases, these data also reflect common clinical experience. It is reasonable to anticipate that this trend toward a decreased incidence of involved pelvic lymph nodes will continue in the future as serial PSA testing becomes a more common means of detection of PCa. As the yield of abnormal lymph nodes has decreased, the emphasis on surgical staging of the lymph nodes has diminished.

PATIENT SELECTION FOR PELVIC LYMPH NODE DISSECTION

It is well established that histologic grade, clinical stage, and PSA level are valuable prognostic factors. Historically, these variables have been examined separately for their ability to predict which patients may have positive lymph nodes. Recently, several studies have attempted to combine these variables to provide a better discrimination of patients who would be unlikely to have metastases in the lymph nodes and thus could be spared a PLND.[7–11] Probability tables have been established that define the risk utilizing grade, clinical stage, and PSA level. Partin et al.,[7] Bishoff et al.,[11] and Sands et al.[10] have established nomograms that allow relatively easy reference to the probability of nodal metastases given a specific clinical scenario (Figs. 8.1, 8.2 and Table 8.1). Then, depending on the threshold rate that one would accept for missing a lymph node metastasis, the surgeon

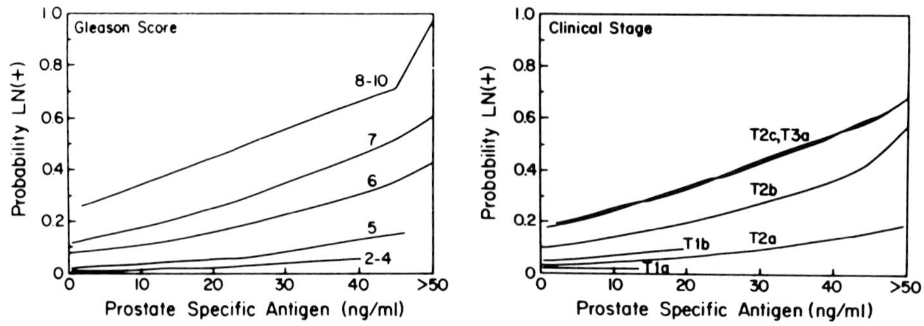

Fig. 8.1. Probability of lymph nodal involvement (LN+) as function of serum PSA and either Gleason score or clinical stage. Reproduced from Partin et al., ref. 7, with permission.

can decide if a PLND is worth the time, effort, and morbidity. Bishoff et al. felt that if a 3% probability of missing positive lymph nodes was acceptable, 37% of patients would not require a PLND; if a 5% probability was accepted, 50% of patients could be spared the dissection.[11] There is no consensus on the appropriate threshold for an acceptable probability of missing an involved node.

It is clear that the trend toward the detection of smaller PCa will only continue. The vast majority of these patients will be at a very low risk for nodal spread and thus PLND will be of little benefit. With a retropubic approach, the additional risk or cost of a PLND is not large but it also may not be trivial. A few patients do have morbidity that may be attributable to the PLND such as prolonged lymph leak, lymphocele, vascular injury, or obturator nerve injury (Fig. 8.3). Also, even if the dissection only adds 30 minutes to the operative time, this may be important in an era of strict cost containment or capitated reimbursement systems. For those surgeons who favor a perineal approach for a RP, the elimination of the PLND may provide a considerable benefit by omitting a separate pro-

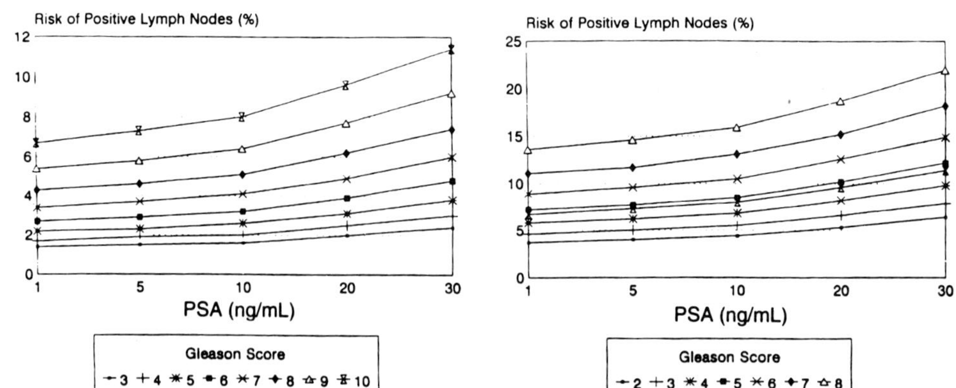

Fig. 8.2. Risk of positive lymph nodes in patients with T2a–b (*left*) or T2c (*right*) prostate cancer by biopsy grade (Gleason total score) and PSA. Reproduced from Bishoff et al., ref. 11, with permission.

TABLE 8.1. Incidence* of Nodal Metastasis According to Stage, Gleason Grade, and PSA Level Based on Multivariate Logistic Regression

		Gleason Grade			
Stage	*PSA (ng/ml)*	*2–4*	*5, 6*	*7*	*8–10*
A2	≤4	<1	1	1	5
	>4 ≤20	1	5	10	15
	>20 ≤40	1	10	15	20
	>40	5	25	35	45
B	≤4	1	5	5	10
	>4 ≤20	5	15	25	35
	>20 ≤40	5	20	35	45
	>40	20	50	65	75
C	≤4	5	10	15	25
	>4 ≤20	10	35	50	60
	>20 ≤40	15	45	60	70
	>40	45	75	85	90

*Incidences are rounded to the nearest 5%.
Reproduced from Sands et al., ref. 10.

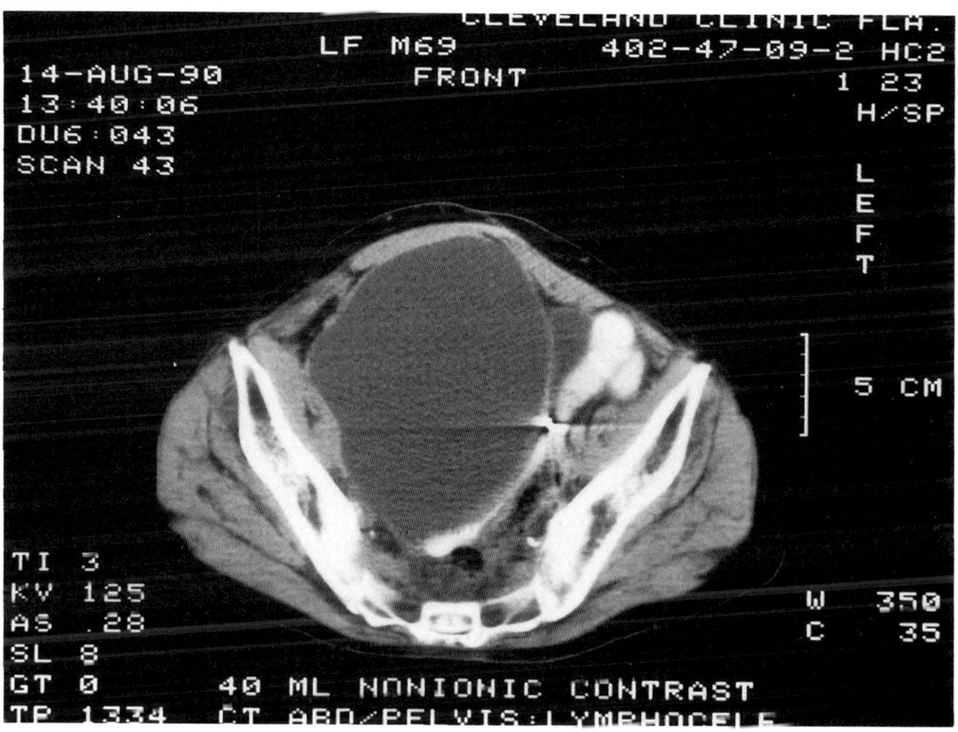

Fig. 8.3. Pelvic lymphocele after pelvic lymphadenectomy demonstrated by CT scan of pelvis.

cedure. Although not widely accepted in clinical practice in 1995, elimination of the PLND in many patients will be common in the future.

METHODS TO DETECT PELVIC LYMPH NODE METASTASES

It is accepted that the first echelon "landing zone" of nodal metastases from PCa is a well-defined anatomic area in the pelvis. Although the anatomic descriptors used to label the nodes have been a source of some confusion, the nodes of interest are intimately associated with the internal and external iliac vessels and the obturator nerve. Imaging studies have not proven to be particularly helpful in the detection of pelvic node metastases. Most nodal metastases are of microscopic size and thus undetected by either pelvic computed tomography (CT) or magnetic resonance imaging. A patient with a substantially elevated PSA, such as >30 ng/ml, may have grossly enlarged pelvic nodes and thus imaging studies may be worthwhile. If enlarged nodes are visualized, it is wise to confirm the presence of metastases with an aspiration biopsy.[12]

A diagnostic PLND attempts to remove or sample the nodes most likely to be involved in early lymphatic spread. Initially, a PLND for PCa included a lymphatic tissue around both the external iliac artery and vein; later, a "modified" dissection was adopted that established the external iliac vein as the lateral limit (Fig. 8.4A–C). There did not appear to be an important decrease in the frequency of identification of involved nodes as the dissection area was decreased and the risk for lymphedema of the genitalia was diminished. Some studies did identify that "hypogastric" nodes associated with the internal iliac artery or presciatic area may harbor metastases when other nodes were negative; however

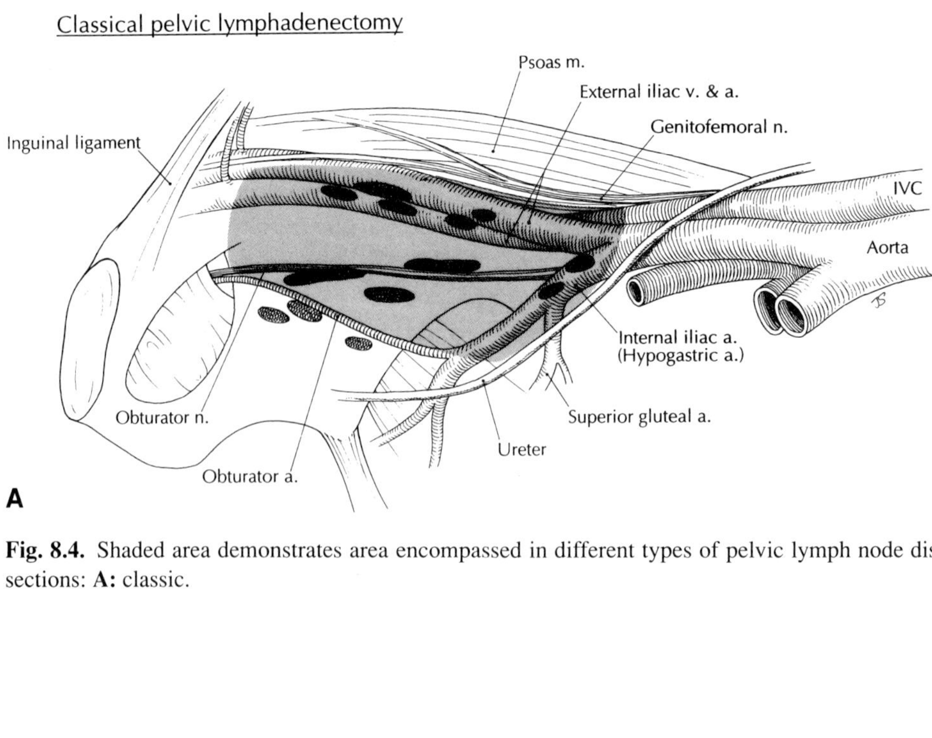

Fig. 8.4. Shaded area demonstrates area encompassed in different types of pelvic lymph node dissections: **A:** classic.

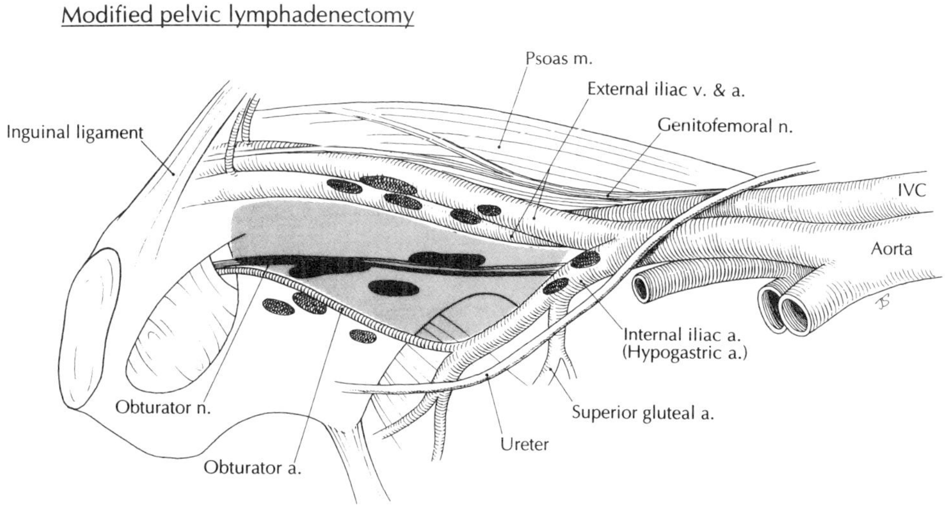

B

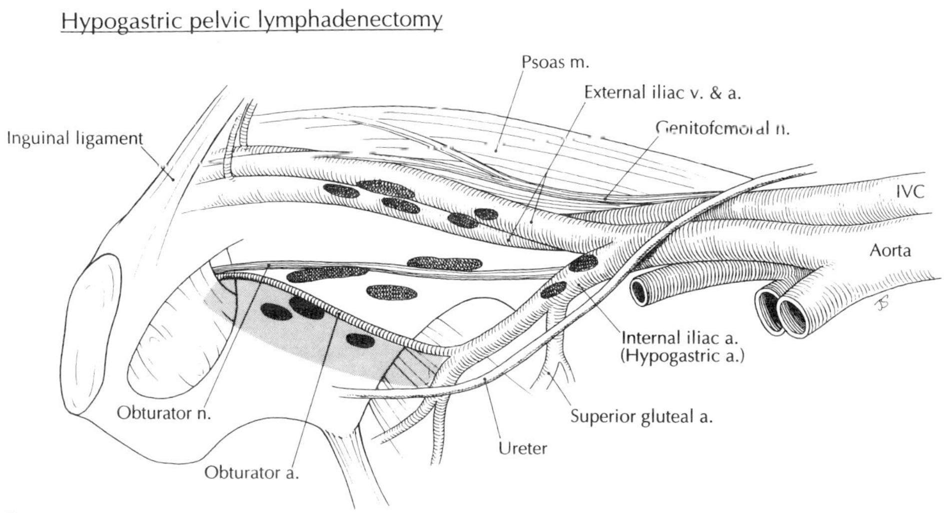

C

Fig. 8.4. B: modified; **C:** hypogastric (presciatic).

this circumstance is uncommon and thus these deeper pelvic nodes are not included in a typical dissection.[2,13] Most surgeons employ the modified dissection to provide a representative sampling of the nodes with minimal morbidity. A therapeutic benefit has not been demonstrated and is not anticipated. Often only a few nodes that are confluent rather than discreet are obtained; resection of additional tissue between the external iliac artery and vein can increase the number of nodes removed but it may not increase the yield of abnormal findings.

Among other factors, the opportunity to easily include a PLND with RP led to the resurgence of popularity of a retropubic approach. As discussed earlier, the finding of a positive node led to the abandonment of the RP. However, if information on the lymph nodes was desired prior to RT, a separate surgical procedure was necessary with attendant morbidity and expense. In this context, the development of a laparoscopic PLND in the late 1980s provided a means to assess the pelvic nodes with apparently less morbidity.[14] As experience with this procedure has increased, the complication rate has decreased and confidence in the completeness of dissection has improved.[15,16] The operation remains in the domain of the limited number of urologists skilled in laparoscopy. Because of the expertise and expense associated with a laparoscopic PLND, some surgeons have advocated an open procedure with a limited incision and dissection, termed a *mini-laparotomy*, with claimed similar results of short hospital stay and quick recovery.[17] To add an additional variable, an extraperitoneal laparoscopic approach is generating interest in an effort to further decrease morbidity.[18]

In summary, there are now four approaches to PLND: classical open dissection, mini-laparotomy, intraperitoneal laparoscopic, and extraperitoneal laparoscopic. There is no reason to believe that node retrieval is inferior with any approach by experienced surgeons. Comparative cost and morbidity data that would infer a particular approach should be exclusively adopted are not available.

On the horizon are several technical advances that may improve identification of patients with PCa metastatic to pelvic lymph nodes. First, a radiolabeled monoclonal antibody to an apparent specific prostate antigen has entered clinical trials.[19] The antibody, CYT-356, when radiolabeled with ^{111}In, theoretically provides an opportunity to specifically detect PCa metastases on a radionuclide scan. While demonstrating some promise in early trials, the imaging is obscure with considerable background uptake in the pelvic vessels and difficulty in the identification of only microscopic or even gross nodal disease might be anticipated.

Another strategy to improve the value of PLND is to better identify true "micrometastasis" in the nodes that might be undetected with traditional sampling and histologic examination. One method capitalizes on the relatively specific staining of epithelial cancer cells with anticytokeratin antibody immunostaining; tiny amounts of cancer cells are more readily identified because of differential staining compared to the normal lymphatic cells in the nodes. While this technique has been valuable in other cancers, preliminary studies in PCa have not detected occult metastases commonly in nodes negative by traditional methods.[20,21] A remarkably sensitive technique is emerging which allows the opportunity to detect messenger RNA from PSA producing cells.[22] Utilizing reverse transcriptase–polymerase chain reaction (RT-PCR) methods, as little as one cancer cell in 1,000,000 lymphoid cells may be detected. The prognostic significance of these truly micrometastases remains to be determined and the assumption cannot be uncritically accepted that all of the patients with the earliest nodal spread will develop systemic spread. Extended follow-up and multivariate comparison with other known prognostic factors will be necessary.

OUTCOME OF THERAPY FOR NODE-POSITIVE PATIENTS

PCa is noteworthy for extremely responsive but noncurative systemic therapy. No other solid tumor demonstrates the endocrine sensitivity that PCa does. Even in patients with bone metastases, 60–80% of men will demonstrate improvement after androgen deprivation and approximately 10% will live 10 years. For the patient with only nodal metastases, complete and partial responses are seen with at least a similar frequency to those with spread limited to the bone.[23] There are some data to support that patients with only nodal disease have a better 5-year survival after endocrine therapy than those with bone metastases.[24] For the patient with grossly evident pelvic or nonregional nodal metastases, there is little debate that initial endocrine therapy is the treatment of choice. RP is not considered; RT may be used for additional palliation of local symptoms. Endocrine therapy may be in the form of traditional monotherapy with an orchiectomy, LH-RH agonist, or estrogens. Combined androgen blockade, i.e., the addition of an antiandrogen in combination with suppression of testicular androgen production, is of uncertain value in this particular setting of only nodal metastases. Whether this patient population with nodal only spread is equivalent to those in the "minimal" disease category for bone metastases and thus potentially more likely to have a substantial benefit from combined therapy is unknown.[25]

The therapeutic decisions about the patient with small-volume nodal metastases identified at the time of PLND remain controversial, regardless of whether RP or RT was planned. There are several issues evident in recent years which have modified the strategies from those widely adopted in the 1980s.

1. Patients with early nodal metastases identified with traditional histologic methods probably all fail based on the presence of a detectable and rising PSA. However, the time for the PSA to become detectable may be protracted, often 3 to 5 years. The lead time from when the PSA becomes detectable until clinically apparent disease is evident on imaging studies may be an additional 3 to 7 years.[26] The time to symptomatic recurrence will be even longer. Thus it is not surprising that even though the patient may die from his PCa, it can easily take 5 to 10 years for this to happen. For the majority of that time, the patient is asymptomatic from the PCa.[27,28] It is important to instill in the patient a positive attitude during this period of freedom from clinical disease so that his anxiety does not interfere with his opportunity to enjoy a near normal lifestyle. Some patients are overwhelmed by the possibility of the "hopelessness" of the situation if positive nodes are found, especially if local therapy is withheld because there was no possibility of "cure." This attitude can be very destructive for a patient and his family and can be engendered by the approach adopted by the physician.

2. Because patients may live for many years even in the face of nodal metastases, there is a possibility of progressive local disease contributing to symptoms during this 5- to 10-year period. Data on symptom progression in the current era is scant. Most local symptoms are controlled by endocrine therapy but not all. Bosch and Schroder found that 10 of 21 men with T3N+ PCa still needed at least one transurethral resection later.[29] Many patients in the setting require repeated surgery to relieve outlet obstruction and thus run further risk of incontinence from the surgery and disease involving the external sphincter. Ureteral obstruction from progressive local disease over many years is also a risk. External radiation may also provide reasonable palliation later if needed but may be less effective as the disease has become bulkier. Prevention of these later local symptoms over time is a rationale for more aggressive local treatment such as RP or RT initially when the local disease is small.[29–31] Management strategies in the urologic community are quite diverse, reflecting the paucity of data to guide treatment decisions.

3. The impact of aggressive local therapy and early endocrine therapy has gained increasing support in recent years. Much of this has been fueled by reports from the Mayo Clinic suggesting extended disease-free intervals in many patients treated by RP and immediate endocrine therapy.[32] The benefit appears to be largely confined to those men with diploid cancers and it is uncertain if there is benefit to the entire group when treated in this fashion. With the strategy of RP and early endocrine therapy in the patients with diploid cancers, cancer deaths before 10 years were rare. The rationale for this approach is treatment of the cancer when it is predominantly diploid and likely to respond well to androgen deprivation rather than later when recurrence is widespread and the cancer is less likely to be diploid. Earlier Veterans Administration Cooperative Group studies demonstrate a benefit of delaying cancer deaths with earlier endocrine therapy in men with metastatic disease; the cancer death rate is also decreased but the overall survival was not changed because of excessive deaths caused by estrogen toxicity.[33] Extrapolation of these data to the setting of patients with positive nodes is tempting but unproven. On a practical basis in the PSA era, most patients are uncomfortable with only observation if a continually rising PSA is present and often desire early endocrine therapy. A more timely question now is the relative benefit of "earliest" endocrine therapy (high-risk because positive nodes were found after RP) versus "earlier" endocrine treatment (PSA begins to rise) versus "early" endocrine treatment (clinically apparent metastatic disease) versus "late" treatment (symptomatic metastasis). "Earliest" treatment is not without morbidity and expense. In addition to near universal impotence and diminished libido, a decrease in vigor and exercise tolerance is common and may interfere with continuing a usual lifestyle. In addition, the consensus practice of continuous hormonal therapy until death may not be necessary or ideal; intermittent hormonal therapy may be particularly well suited to study in this specific group of patients who have no detectable disease other than an elevated PSA.

4. The relative contribution of aggressive local therapy in the face of involved pelvic lymph nodes remains the most controversial aspect of the clinical situation. The patient has systemic disease, local therapy has side effects and will not effect the outcome, so why give it? Could comparable results be obtained with just the endocrine therapy, reserving local therapy such as a transurethral resection of the prostate or palliative RT for those who develop symptomatic local progression? The questions cannot presently be answered conclusively. However, the best reported results have been with a combination of RP and immediate hormonal therapy.[32,34–36] Undoubtedly, patient selection factors may contribute to these favorable results.[28,37]

In my opinion, there are intangible factors that may influence treatment decisions in individual patients.[38] Most patients with localized prostate cancer become extremely well-informed about treatment options and actively participate in the decision about which treatment to receive. Once the patient has made the decision to have a RP over other treatment options, they perceive of this as the preferred therapy. Patients then being told that the presence of an involved lymph node precludes them from having this preferred therapy are commonly devastated; reestablishing a positive attitude toward their treatment with a goal of enjoying their remaining life is often difficult. They perceive the situation as near hopeless, when the reality is that they will often have an extended period of many years when they are essentially asymptomatic. The key variable in this dilemma is the morbidity of the surgery. If we subject the patient to a RP in the face of an involved node and the patient becomes incontinent after surgery, we have actually worsened his quality of life for his remaining years. The patient has the worst of both worlds, i.e., failure of cure and morbidity from the treatment. If RP had no potential for severe side effects, this debate would largely disappear. Clearly, no single "right" answer exists. However, a stronger trend is evident in our practice and in many other academic centers to proceed with the RP unless the lymph nodes are grossly involved with the anticipation of a low morbidity from the surgery and adjuvant endocrine therapy in an effort to provide as long a disease-free interval as possible. This approach certainly cannot be considered ideal for all patients and is subject to reevaluation as more data become available.

REFERENCES

1. Smith JA Jr, Seaman JP, Gleidman JB, et al: Pelvic lymph node metastasis from prostatic cancer: influence of tumor grade and stage in 452 consecutive patients. *J Urol* 130:290–292, 1983.
2. McDowell GC II, Johnson JW, Tenney DM, et al: Pelvic lymphadenectomy for staging clinically localized prostate cancer. *Urology* 35(6):476–482, 1990.
3. Fowler JE Jr, Whitmore WF Jr: The incidence and extent of pelvic lymph node metastases in apparently localized prostatic cancer. *Cancer* 47(12):2941–2945, 1981.
4. Catalona WJ: Screening for prostate cancer: enthusiasm. *Urology* 42(2):113–115, 1993.
5. Petros JA, Catalona WJ: Lower incidence of unsuspected lymph node metastases in 521 consecutive patients with clinically localized prostate cancer. *J Urol* 147:1574–1575, 1992.
6. Danella JF, deKernion JB, Smith RB, et al: The contemporary incidence of lymph node metastases in prostate cancer: implications for laparoscopic lymph node dissection. *J Urol* 149:1488–1491, 1993.
7. Partin AW, Yoo J, Carter HB, et al: The use of prostate specific antigen, clinical stage, and Gleason score to predict pathologic stage in men with localized prostate cancer. *J Urol* 150:110–114, 1993.
8. Wolf JS Jr, Perinchery N, Shinohara K, et al: Selection of patients for laparoscopic pelvic lymphadenectomy prior to radical prostatectomy: a decision analysis. *Urology* 42(6):680–688, 1993.
9. Blackwell KL, Bostwick DG, Myers RP, et al: Combining prostate specific antigen with cancer and gland volume to predict more reliably pathological stage: the influence of prostate specific antigen cancer density. *J Urol* 151:1565–1570, 1994.
10. Sands ME, Zagars GK, Pollack A, et al: Serum prostate-specific antigen, clinical stage, pathologic grade, and the incidence of nodal metastases in prostate cancer. *Urology* 44(2):215–220, 1994.
11. Bishoff JT, St Clair SR, Reyes A, et al: Pelvic lymphadenectomy can be omitted in selected patients with carcinoma of the prostate: development of a system of patient selection. *Urology* 45(2):270–274, 1995.
12. Flanigan RC, Mohler JL, King CT, et al: Preoperative lymph node evaluation in prostatic cancer patients who are surgical candidates: the role of lymphangiography and computerized tomography scanning with directed fine needle aspiration. *J Urol* 134:84–87, 1985.
13. Golimbu M, Morales P: Extended pelvic lymphadenectomy. *Urology* 15(3):298–301, 1980.
14. Kerbl K, Clayman RV, Petros JA: Staging pelvic lymphadenectomy for prostate cancer: a comparison of laparoscopic and open techniques. *J Urol* 150:396–399, 1993.

15. Kavoussi LR, Sosa E, Chandhoke P, et al: Complications of laparoscopic pelvic lymph node dissection. *J Urol* 149:322–325, 1993.
16. Guazzoni G, Montorsi F, Bergamaschi F, et al: Open surgical revision of laparoscopic pelvic lymphadenectomy for staging of prostate cancer: the impact of laparoscopic learning curve. *J Urol* 151:930–933, 1994.
17. Steiner MS, Marshall FF: Mini-laparotomy staging pelvic lymphadenectomy (minilap). *Urology* 41(3):201–206, 1993.
18. Das S, Tashima M: Extraperitoneal laparoscopic staging pelvic lymph node dissection. *J Urol* 151:1321–1323, 1994.
19. Murphy GP: Radioscintiscanning of prostate cancer. *Cancer* (Suppl) 75(7):1819–1822, 1995.
20. Gomella LG, White JL, McCue PA, et al: Screening for occult nodal metastasis in localized carcinoma of the prostate. *J Urol* 149:776–778, 1993.
21. Moul JW, Kahn DG, Lewis DJ, et al: Immunohistologic detection of prostate cancer pelvic lymph node micrometastases: correlation to preoperative serum prostate-specific antigen. *Urology* 43(1):68–73, 1994.
22. Deguchi T, Doi T, Ehara H, et al: Detection of micrometastatic prostate cancer cells in lymph nodes by reverse transcriptase–polymerase chain reaction. *Cancer Res* 53:5350–5354, 1993.
23. Saeter G, Fossa SD, Ous S, et al: Carcinoma of the prostate with soft tissue or non-regional lymphatic metastases at the time of diagnosis: a review of 47 cases. *Br J Urol* 56:385–390, 1984.
24. Sandhu DPS, Mayor PE, Sambrook P, et al: Increased survival of patients with massive lymphadenopathy and prostate cancer: evidence of heterogeneous tumour behaviour. *Br J Urol* 66:415–419, 1990.
25. Crawford ED, Eisenberger MA, McLeod DG, et al: A controlled trial of leuprolide with and without flutamide in prostatic carcinoma. *N Engl J Med* 321(7):419–424, 1989.
26. Montie JE: Follow-up after radical prostatectomy or radiation therapy for prostate cancer. *Urol Clin North Am* 21(4):673–676, 1994.
27. Kramolowsky EV: The value of testosterone deprivation in stage D1 carcinoma of the prostate. *J Urol* 139:1242–1244, 1988.
28. Frazier HA II, Robertson JE, Paulson DF: Does radical prostatectomy in the presence of positive pelvic lymph nodes enhance survival? *World J Urol* 12:308–312, 1994.
29. Bosch R, Schroder FH: Radical prostatectomy and adjuvant endocrine treatment: a review. *Prog Clin Biol Res* 359:239–247, 1990.
30. Steinberg GD, Epstein JI, Piantadosi S, et al: Management of stage D1 adenocarcinoma of the prostate: the Johns Hopkins experience 1974 to 1987. *J Urol* 144:1425–1432, 1990.
31. Lawton CA, Cox JD, Glisch C, et al: Is long-term survival possible with external beam irradiation for stage D1 adenocarcinoma of the prostate? *Cancer* 69(11):2761–2766, 1992.
32. Zincke H: The role of pathologic variables and hormonal treatment after radical prostatectomy for stage D1 disease. *Oncology* 5(3):129–139, 1991.
33. Byar DP, Corle DK: Hormone therapy for prostate cancer: results of the Veterans Administration Cooperative Urological Research Group studies. *NCI Monographs* 7:165–170, 1988.
34. deKernion JB, Neuwirth H, Stein A, et al: Prognosis of patients with stage D1 prostate carcinoma following radical prostatectomy with and without early endocrine therapy. *J Urol* 144:700–703, 1990.
35. Zagars GK, Sands ME, Pollack A, et al: Early androgen ablation for stage D1 (N1 to N3, MO) prostate cancer: prognostic variables and outcome. *J Urol* 151:1330–1333, 1994.

36. Freeman JA, Cook DW, Lieskovsky G, et al: Adjuvant radiation, chemotherapy, and androgen deprivation therapy for pathologic stage D1 adenocarcinoma of the prostate. *Urology* 44(5):719–725, 1994.

37. Sgrignoli AR, Walsh PC, Steinberg GD, et al: Prognostic factors in men with stage D1 prostate cancer: identification of patients less likely to have prolonged survival after radical prostatectomy. *J Urol* 152:1077–1081, 1994.

38. Montie JE: Counseling the patient with regional metastasis of prostate cancer. *Cancer* (Suppl) 71(3):1019–1023, 1993.

9

Treatment of Locally Extensive But Nonmetastatic Prostate Cancer (Stage C)

Thomas A. Rozanski
Ian M. Thompson

Locally advanced carcinoma of the prostate (stage C, or T3) includes all conditions in which tumor extends beyond the confines of the gland but is not fixed to pelvic structures. Several staging systems exist which subclassify T3 disease. The American Joint Committee on Cancer and the International Union Against Cancer staging system classifies T3a disease as unilateral extracapsular extension, T3b as bilateral extracapsular extension, and tumor invading the seminal vesicles as T3c. Some authors include in the T3a category any surgical specimen with tumor invading or penetrating the capsule with clear surgical margins, while T3b describes tumor at the surgical margin.

The incidence of T3 disease decreased between 1974 (17.7%) and 1983 (12.3%) in American College of Surgeons (ACS) surveys.[1] This stage migration was probably due to the increased use of bone scintigraphy which excluded patients with bony metastases. However, by 1991, T3 disease represented 18.5% of prostate cancers.[2] This increase corresponds to the sharp rise in the rate of radical prostatectomy for localized disease, and may represent an increase in capsular penetration or margin positive disease, not bulky T3 disease. This migration to lower clinical stages most likely reflects the routine use of both prostate specific antigen (PSA) and digital rectal examination (DRE). Unfortunately, clinical staging is inaccurate; approximately 30% to 60% of men thought clinically to have organ-confined disease and treated with prostatectomy, will have pathologic T3 (pT3) disease.[3,4] The increase in pT3 disease may be the result of more complete, whole-mount histologic examinations of prostatectomy specimens. Approximately 19% of men found to have cancer in screening programs will have T3 disease.[4,5]

Clinical staging of prostate cancer is difficult. Up to 60% of clinical T2 tumors will have extension of tumor beyond the gland. Conversely, historical data suggest that 4% to 30% of clinical T3 disease is overstaged and truly represents organ-confined tumor at prostatectomy.[6–9] It is not known to what degree overstaging occurs in men who have undergone radical prostatectomy for T3 disease who are evaluated by contemporary extensive pathologic techniques. When DRE is suspicious for gross extension of tumor beyond the gland, the vast majority of these patients will have at least T3 disease. Forty-two to 56% of patients thought to have clinical T3 disease will have tumor in pelvic lymph nodes at exploration.[6,10–12] PSA values are not helpful in differentiating those patients with nodal metastasis. Greskovich found that the mean PSA was virtually identical in patients with C and D1 disease.[11] The use of imaging modalities for clinical staging has little benefit in improving the diagnosis of pathologic C disease. The sensitivities of transrectal ultrasound (TRUS), computed tomography (CT), and magnetic resonance imaging (MRI) are 66%, 55%, and 77% respectively, while specificity is only 46%, 65%, and 57%.[13,14] The overall staging accuracy of endorectal surface coil MRI is 68%, the majority of failures being microscopic extracapsular disease.[15] A much higher accuracy (91%) is reported for depicting seminal vesicle involvement, however, when compared to whole-mount pathologic specimens, endorectal coil MRI is not helpful in staging.[15,16] Cummings and colleagues reported on the value of TRUS in preoperatively detecting seminal vesicle tumor invasion.[17] They found that a total seminal vesicle volume greater than 15 cc and asymmetry of the seminal vesicles strongly suggested T3c disease (B1).

The biochemical diagnosis of T3 disease using either PSA or prostatic acid phosphatase (PAP) is unreliable. While PSA has had a marked effect on the diagnosis and follow-up of patients with prostate cancer, the test has poor specificity for detecting local extension of tumor beyond the gland. PAP is rarely used today as it adds little beyond routine staging. The only specific area in which the enzymatic PAP assay is superior to PSA is the preoperative evaluation for extracapsular tumor. PAP specificity for extracapsular disease is high, unfortunately the sensitivity is very low and therefore PAP does not identify most patients with incurable disease. In addition, the vast majority of patients with T3 disease and an elevated PAP also have very suggestive DRE, and PSA values are usually over 100 ng/ml.[18] Burnett et al. estimated that PAP contributes unique information in only 1% of patients.[19]

The long-term outlook for men diagnosed with stage T3 carcinoma of the prostate is poor. The aggressive nature of T3 tumors may be due to aggressive biologic activity, since the tumor has already demonstrated its ability for local metastasis. This is quite evident from the higher tumor grade noted in patients with T3 disease (Table 9.1). DNA ploidy features may also contribute to the malignant course of T3 disease. Several investigators have shown that stage C tumors have a higher degree of aneuploidy than stage A and B tumors.[20,21]

Recurrent disease and survival differ for the subcategories of T3 disease. Schellhammer noted that patients with seminal vesicle tumor invasion had an increased rate of local and distant failures compared to patients with capsular extension only.[22] Epstein et al. reported that progression-free survival was decreased in patients with extensive capsular penetration when compared to men with focal capsular penetration.[23] Since patients with seminal vesicle invasion have such a poor prognosis, some advocate seminal vesicle biopsy prior to instituting curative treatments. In a group of patients with clinically localized prostate cancer, 16.5% were found to have a positive seminal vesicle biopsy prior to radical prostatectomy.[24] When compared to prostatectomy specimens, the positive predictive value of a preoperative seminal vesicle biopsy was 100%, and negative predictive value was 87.5%. Tumor invasion of the seminal vesicles was associated with larger tumor volumes, a fourfold increase in positive surgical margins, and a threefold increase in capsular perforation. In addition, patients with seminal vesicle disease had greater local

TABLE 9.1. Grade Distribution of Prostate Cancer by Stage

	Clinical Stage			
Tumor Grade	*T1a*	*T1b–c*	*T2*	*T3–4*
Well	25.5	34.8	27.5	12.2
Moderately–well	1.6	30.5	35.2	32.7
Poor	1.6	16.6	24.3	57.5

From Mettlin, ref. 2.

recurrence and diminished interval to recurrence. Given the bleak outlook for patients with pT3c tumors, high-risk patients may deserve additional biopsies before initiating therapy.

Survival statistics for various treatment options offered to patients with T3 disease are often difficult to compare. A wide variety of treatments have been employed, including curative and noncurative regimens, and single or combination therapies. An obvious selection bias exists in those treated with aggressive attempts for cure. Historical controls are often inadequate since PSA and bone scan were not routinely used until recently, allowing patients with unrecognized lymphatic and bony metastases to be staged as C disease. Early biochemical failures were not recognized until the advent of PSA.

The suboptimal outcomes for patients treated for T3 prostate cancer are reflected in the fact that there is no consensus as to what comprises optimal therapy. There is no gold standard for comparison. In an American College of Surgeons survey published in 1986, 47.7% of patients with stage C tumors were treated with noncurative measures, while 52.3% underwent a variety of treatment regimens for "cure."[1] A more recent review has found an increase in putatively curative treatment yet a wide variation in treatment has been offered for this stage of disease (Fig. 9.1).

TREATMENTS

A review of the literature analyzing the treatment of patients with stage T3 prostate cancer leads to a single conclusion. Any form of monotherapy, be it surgical or radiation, has a low chance of curing the patient.

External Beam Radiotherapy

The modality used most frequently as monotherapy to treat stage T3 prostate cancer has been external beam radiation (XRT). Local control rates vary among series, many are not reported relative to the period of follow-up, and older series do not include PSA or biopsy data. M.D. Anderson reported 10-year local control rates of 79% to 81%[25,26] similar to the 82% reported by Wilson at Yale.[27] Schellhammer reviewed recurrence after XRT for clinical stage C disease with follow-up over 7 years, and local failures ranged from 28% to 36%.[28]

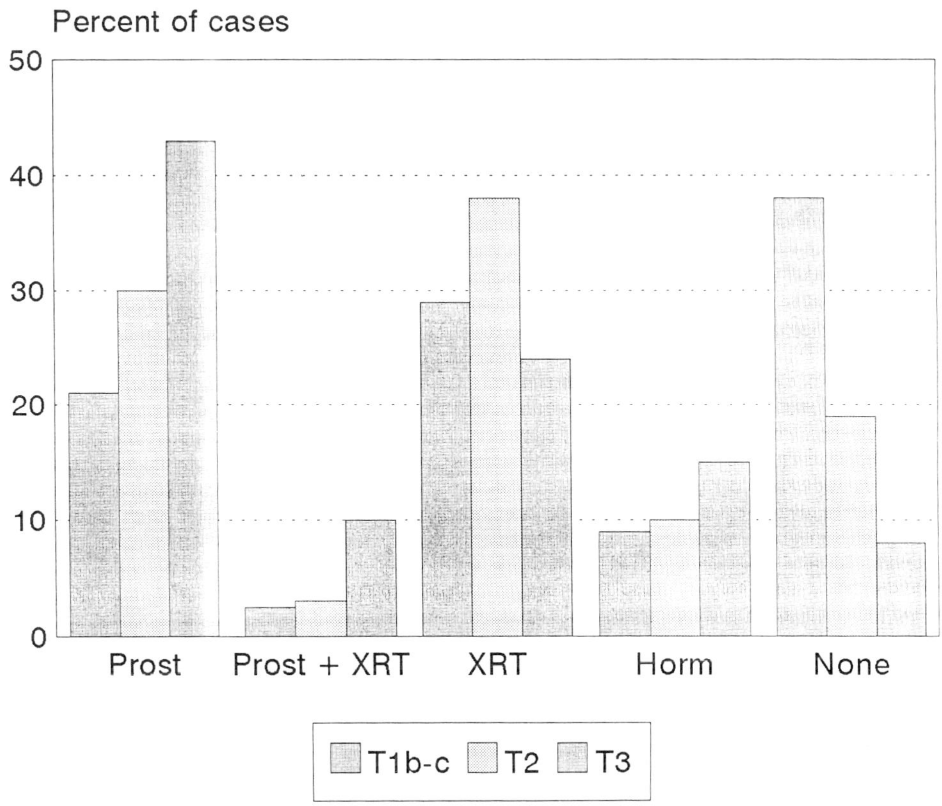

Fig. 9.1. Treatment of prostate cancer by clinical stage, 1994.

Survival rates after definitive radiotherapy vary considerably. Caution must be exercised to compare similar survival definitions, i.e., metastatic-free survival, cancer-specific survival, disease-free survival, overall survival, etc. as the ascertainment of all but the last of these can be quite variable. Overall survival data on over 3,000 patients in 21 series shows 5-, 10-, and 15-year rates of 63%, 39%, and 24%.[29] Disease-free survival rates must be regarded with scrutiny since historical data do not include PSA-only failures. M.D. Anderson reported in 1994 that 62% of patients with stage C disease treated by XRT developed relapse or a rising PSA at 5 years.[30] Corn and associates in 1995 reported that only 41% of patients with T3 disease treated with definitive radiation were free of progression at 3 years follow-up.[31] Whereas prostatectomy series consider any measurable PSA as a failure, radiation oncologists are not in agreement and values ranging from less than 1.0 to 4.0 ng/ml have been considered consistent with cure or control. Controversy also surrounds postradiation biopsies. In the 1980s, positive biopsies after XRT were reported in up to 74% of patients using conventional biopsy techniques.[32] Recently, TRUS-guided multiple biopsies in patients judged to have a satisfactory clinical response after XRT, demonstrated positive biopsies in 92%.[33] The likelihood of finding a positive biopsy probably depends on how vigorously the biopsy and interpretation are performed.

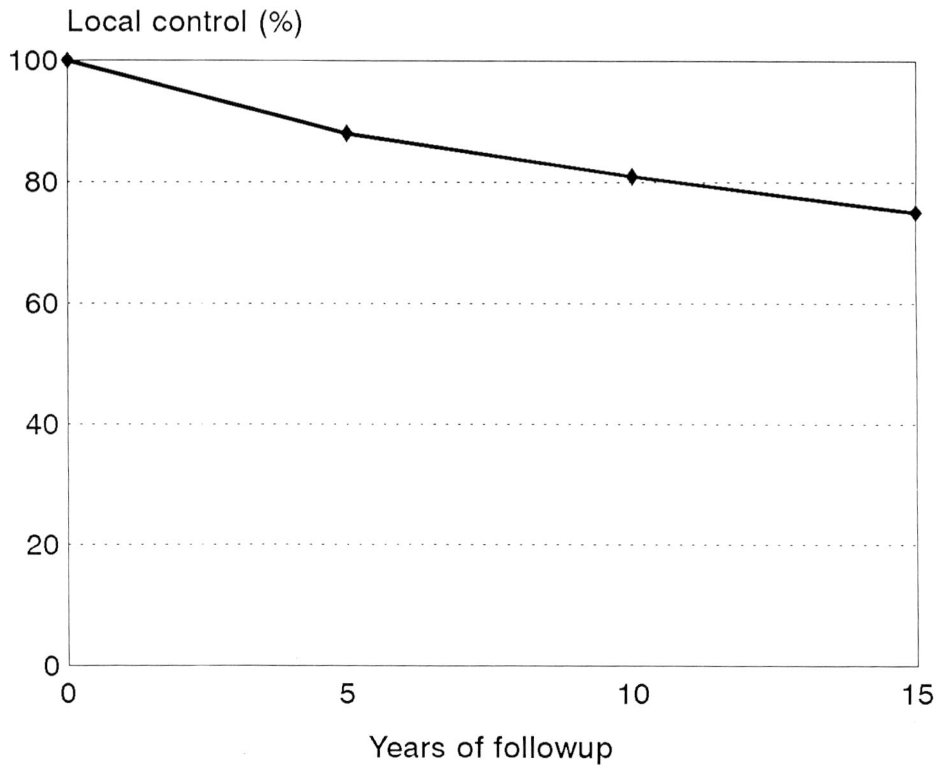

Fig. 9.2. Local control rate with external beam radiation therapy.

Failures are statistically higher in patients with a positive biopsy obtained 18 months or longer after XRT. However, Schellhammer reported 4 of 22 (18%) patients who had a positive biopsy after XRT who remain clinically free of disease for more than 10 years.[28] Examples of local control, actuarial survival, and disease-free survival rates are displayed in Figures 9.2 to 9.4.

Radiation therapy is usually well tolerated and most complications are mild or moderate in severity. Significant complications occur in 6% to 8% of patients.[25] Babian reported that 33% of patients experienced some complication after XRT, and Zagars reported a 34% complication rate, with 3% being of severe degree.[25,26] However, the common complaints of transient acute proctitis and cystitis were not considered complications in these series. Urinary complications, including hematuria, irritation, contracted bladder, ulceration, urethral stricture, and ureteral obstruction occurred in 17% of patients. Three of the 540 evaluable patients required cystectomy and two others urinary diversion.[25] Anorectal complications occurred in 23%, and 12 patients (2%) required a diverting colostomy.[25] Radiation doses above 68 Gy were associated with higher complications. The loss of potency following XRT ranges from 30% to 40%.[34] Overall, though external beam radiotherapy is usually well tolerated, the results of XRT in the treatment of stage T3 carcinoma of the prostate are not encouraging, and long-term cure is unlikely.

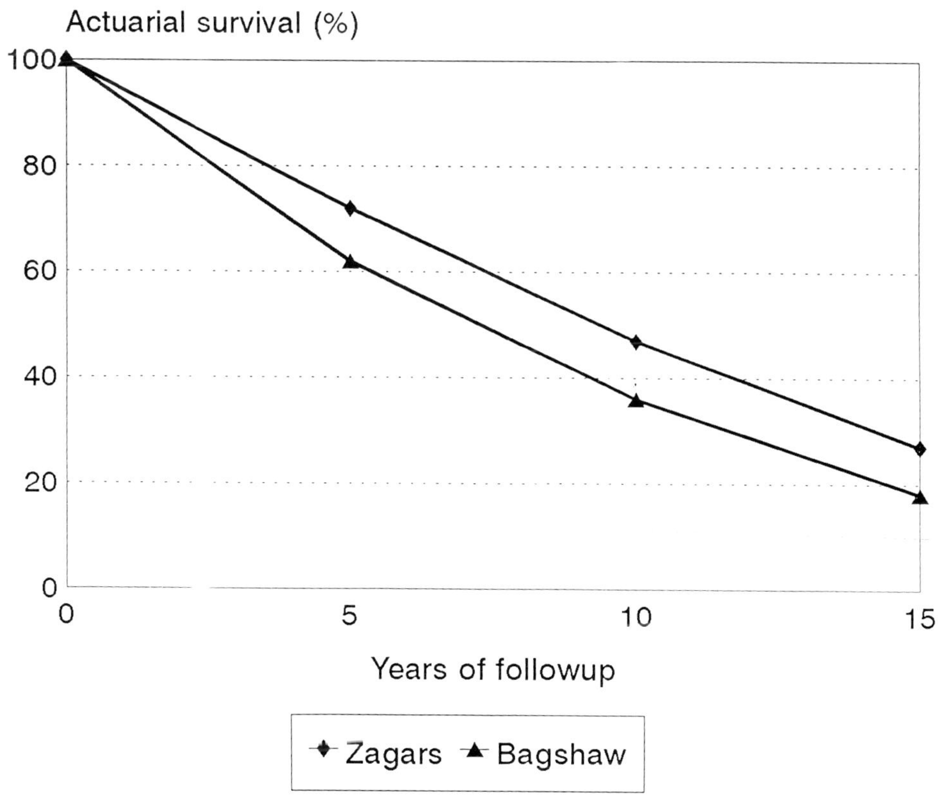

Fig. 9.3. Actuarial survival following external beam radiation therapy.

Brachytherapy

Interstitial radiotherapy for carcinoma of the prostate was popularized in the 1950s using interstitial colloidal gold (^{198}Au). Additional radioactive agents employed include iodine-125, iridium-192, and more recently palladium-103. One oft cited requirement of any form of radiation therapy is the achievement of local control. This intermediate endpoint may help assess the efficacy of treating a disease such as prostate cancer that has a prolonged clinical course. Zagars et al. found that 10-year metastatic-free survival after XRT for prostate cancer was 64% in patients with local disease control compared to only 41% in men who had local recurrence.[35] The Stanford experience was similar with 56% disease-specific survival among patients who achieved local control, compared to 35% in those without local tumor control.[36] Thus, one early indicator of the efficacy of radiotherapy is its ability to achieve local control.

It is in this regard, the ability to achieve local control, that interstitial radiation therapy fails to measure up to external beam therapy. Thompson reviewed several series and found that local control rates with brachytherapy were 15% to 60% lower than seen with XRT.[37] These poor results may translate directly into ultimate patient outcomes. A review of the literature suggests lower overall survival in patients with prostate cancer treated

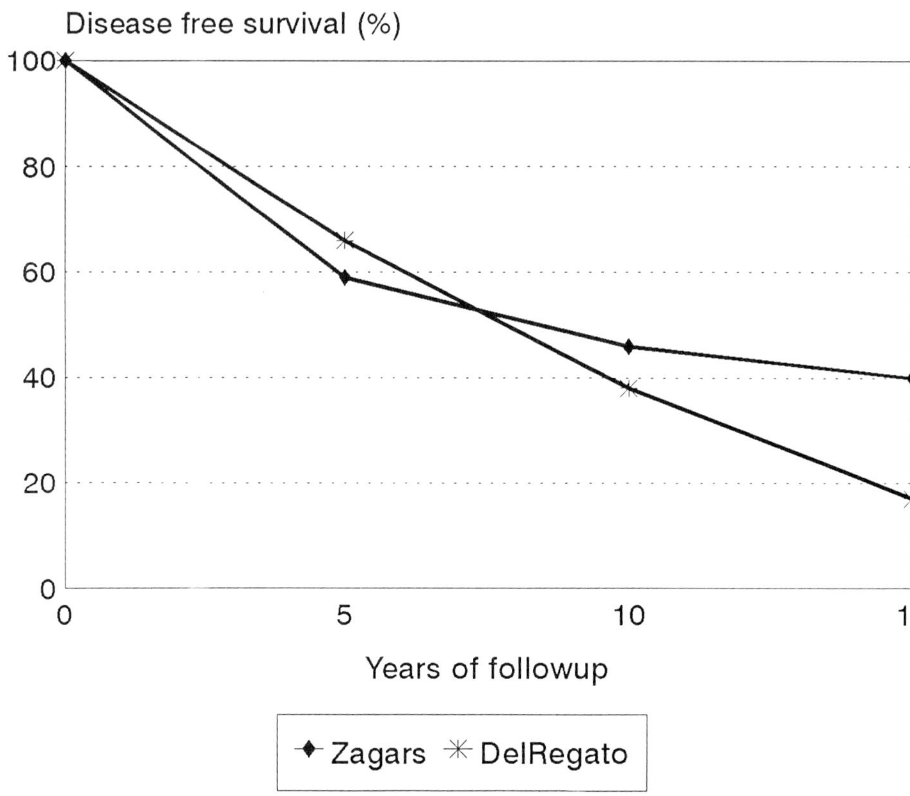

Fig. 9.4. Disease-free survival following external beam radiation therapy.

with interstitial radiation.[29] The morbidity of brachytherapy is higher than that reported with XRT. Holzman and colleagues reported that 60% of patients suffered one or more adverse events, 69% of which were categorized as severe.[38] Kahn reported complications of interstitial ^{192}Ir to treat stage T3 prostate cancer. Toxicity was low with no patients suffering severe or fatal event, however, disease-free survival at 5 years was only 45%.[39]

There has been a recent renewed interest in brachytherapy utilizing ultrasound-guided placement of palladium seeds. Enthusiasm is high among some radiation oncologists, however, firm data are not yet available to compare results with prior radiation series. As yet, no study has shown that interstitial radiation therapy yields better results than external beam radiotherapy.

Radical Prostatectomy

The ideal patients who would benefit from radical prostatectomy are those with organ-confined disease in whom total extirpation of the disease can be accomplished. Therefore, patients with stage T3 tumors are by definition less than ideal candidates. There are few radical prostatectomy series for T3 disease that do not include adjuvant therapy and many series do not differentiate between clinical and pathologic stage T3 disease, causing difficulties in determining the efficacy of radical surgery alone.

Van den Ouden reported on 100 men who underwent radical prostatectomy as monotherapy for clinical stage C tumors. Only 39 patients actually had pathologic T3 disease, 9% were overstaged and found to have pT2 tumors, while 48% had tumor in pelvic lymph nodes.[6] After 4 years of follow-up in the pT3 group, local recurrence developed in 22% and disease progression in 69%. High-grade tumors fared much worse, and when grade 3 tumors were excluded, short-term results were similar to prostatectomy performed for T1 and T2 disease.

A literature review of overall survival in patients with clinical T3 disease who underwent radical prostatectomy showed 5-, 10-, and 15-year survival of 63%, 34%, and 20%, respectively.[29] These data are not significantly different from survival data for similar patients treated with XRT.[29] Exenterative (cystoprostatectomy) procedures for locally extensive prostate cancer have demonstrated no additional efficacy and high morbidity.[29,40] No firm data suggest that radical prostatectomy is superior to XRT in the treatment of stage T3 prostate cancer. Perhaps with the increased numbers of radical prostatectomy being performed for clinically localized disease, long-term follow-up of microscopic stage C tumors will provide important information as to the best therapy for locally advanced prostate cancer.

Cryotherapy

Cryosurgical ablation of the prostate (CSAB) is not a new procedure. The use of subzero temperatures to destroy diseased prostate tissue was described in 1964.[41] Open perineal CSAB for patients with stage C disease was performed in the early 1970s, including patients treated with neoadjuvant hormonal therapy.[42] Bonney reported 5- and 10-year survival rates similar to those achieved with radical prostatectomy at the same institution.[43] Recently there has been a resurgence in enthusiasm for cryosurgery using TRUS percutaneous guidance and urethral warming. Several 3 to 7-mm cryoprobes are positioned in the prostate and liquid nitrogen is placed into the probes, achieving temperatures of −180° to −190°C. Tissue destruction occurs with crystallization and cell membrane rupture, intracellular dehydration, protein denaturation, and thermal shock.[44] Probes can be placed accurately using ultrasound guidance, including placement of probes outside of the gland laterally, and into the seminal vesicles. TRUS monitoring of posterior iceball progression with destruction of prostate tissue and sparing of rectal mucosa is very accurate in the canine model as frozen tissue is clearly distinguished ultrasonographically from nonfrozen tissue.[45] Histologic evaluation shows hemorrhagic infarction.

Miller et al. used CSAB to treat 62 men with clinical stage C prostate cancer between 1990 and 1993.[46] Average hospital stay was 2 days and morbidity was minimal. Prostate biopsies 3 months after CSAB revealed no residual cancer in 79% of patients. The patients with a negative biopsy had a mean PSA of 0.59 ng/ml 3 months after CSAB. These short-term results are encouraging. Formal, well-designed scientific studies need to be performed to assess the long-term efficacy of CSAB. There is presently insufficient evidence that cryosurgery should become standard therapy for stage T3 disease. The American Urological Association Position Statement on Cryoablation was released in August 1993 and the AUA board of directors reaffirmed that position in January 1995: The efficacy of cryoablation for treatment of cancer of the prostate has not yet been established. Its use is considered to be investigational. It is not approved by the Food and Drug Administration for prostate cancer treatment. Cryoablation is, therefore, not recommended for treatment of prostate cancer unless it is part of an approved protocol or controlled regimen of treatment with appropriate full disclosure to the patient.

Conservative Management

Radiotherapy and prostatectomy are rarely curative for stage T3 prostate cancer. Many urologists treat these men with noncurative therapy, primarily hormonal manipulation. Androgen ablation can provide dramatic local responses and prolonged symptomatic improvement.[47] The Veterans Administration Cooperative Urological Research Group (VACURG) showed that androgen deprivation delayed bony metastases in patients with stage C disease, however, overall survival was not affected.[48] Blackard reviewed the data 25 years after the VACURG study and concluded that early endocrine treatment improved quality of life factors.[49] Early hormonal therapy delayed osseous metastases, decreased cancer pain, and improved performance status. Recent evidence suggests that early maximum androgen blockade in patients with metastatic disease and good performance status may increase survival.[50] Early total blockade is probably the treatment of choice if hormonal therapy is considered, unless potency is a major quality of life issue. Fleshner and Trachtenberg reported that of 10 potent patients treated with flutamide and finasteride, eight remained potent, yet mean PSA decreased from 34 to 3.8 ng/ml.[51] This combination may achieve total androgen deprivation with fewer side effects than other combination regimens.

Adolfsson followed 50 patients with low-grade stage C tumors.[52] Delayed hormone therapy was used in 58%. He reported disease-specific survival and overall survival at 5 and 9 years, that is, not significantly different from T3 patients treated with prostatectomy or XRT. Ninety-six percent of his cohort of patients had well to moderately differentiated tumors, while the grade of the majority of T3 disease in most series is moderate to poor. Hanno described no difference in time to the first evidence of distant metastasis in stage T3 patients randomly assigned to either external beam radiotherapy or delayed hormone therapy.[53] A Finnish study with short 4-year follow-up found no difference in progression in patients with locally advanced prostate cancer randomized to orchiectomy, estrogens, or radiotherapy. Orchiectomy had few complications, whereas estrogens and radiation had a high risk of adverse events.[54]

The results of radical surgery and radiation therapy for clinical stage C carcinoma of the prostate differ little from results seen with observation and hormonal therapy alone.[37] Tumor grade and stage, the morbidity and cost of various treatment modalities, and the wishes, expectations, and health of patients should be carefully considered before initiating any form of treatment for stage T3 prostate cancer.

Adjuvant Therapy

Approximately 50% of men undergoing radical prostatectomy for clinically localized disease will have pathologic T3 cancer. Older series on adjuvant radiotherapy following prostatectomy often treated clinically evident disease, and the results of definitive XRT for established local recurrence are disappointing.[55] Currently, biochemical failures using PSA are noted much sooner than the appearance of clinical disease. The Mayo Clinic reported that the efficacy of adjuvant radiation is a strong function of both the PSA level at the time of treatment and the dose of radiation given.[56] Initiating adjuvant radiation when

PSA was greater than 1.0 ng/ml was associated with poor local control. Treating patients with less than 64 Gy resulted in a high failure rate. They concluded that radiation is most effective when the least number of tumor cells exist, and recommend treating patients with adjuvant XRT before PSA rises above 1.0 ng/ml.

McCarthy and coworkers reported on 64 patients who received postoperative XRT for either microscopic T3 disease or a rising PSA.[57] Sixty-seven percent of patients with microscopic T3 tumor had no recurrence at 40 months if radiation was given within the first 6 months after surgery. Sixty-eight percent of men with a delayed rise in PSA treated with adjuvant XRT remained disease-free at 28 months. If measurable PSA values persisted after prostatectomy, 53% of patients treated with XRT initially achieved an undetectable PSA, but a durable response at 3 years occurred in only 33%. They concluded that patients with pT3 disease most likely to benefit from adjuvant radiation are those who have an undetectable PSA after surgery. No difference was noted in patients treated immediately, or if adjuvant therapy was withheld until a rise in PSA was detected. Thompson noted a 50% to 68% failure rate by 3 years in patients treated with adjuvant XRT for a rising PSA after prostatectomy.[58]

Adjuvant XRT seems to decrease local recurrence rates after prostatectomy in patients with pT3 tumors, from 16% to 30% after surgery alone, to 5–8% in the radiated patients at 5 years.[17,29,55] Time to recurrence is increased after adjuvant XRT, but cause-specific and overall survival are not changed.[59] Thompson reported a significant decrease in local failure following adjuvant XRT and an 8% to 9% increase in disease-free survival, however, no change in overall survival at 10 years.[58] The morbidity of adjuvant XRT can be reduced by delaying treatment until continence is restored postoperatively. The value of adjuvant radiation therapy for pathologic T3 disease will be answered definitively by an ongoing randomized trial of radiation versus observation (SWOG 8794, INT 0086). Thus far, this study has randomized 324 of the anticipated 588 patients.

An alternative to adjuvant radiation is postoperative adjuvant hormone therapy. Androgen deprivation has been shown to decrease progression, however, no effect on survival is appreciated.[7] Orchiectomy and XRT have been reported to have similar efficacy in maintaining local control after prostatectomy in stage C patients.[59] The risks and costs of adjuvant treatment should be considered, and eligible patients should be encouraged to participate in formal protocols.

Neoadjuvant Hormone Therapy

Clinical T1–T2 Disease

Radical prostatectomy is currently the most common form of therapy for clinically localized prostate cancer. Despite improvements in clinical staging and a stage migration towards smaller tumors, a significant percentage of men will be found to have extraprostatic tumor after surgery. The finding of pT3 disease portends additional risks for disease recurrence and progression, as well as the risks of additional treatment with its attendant morbidity. A number of investigators have suggested that the incidence of pT3 disease can be reduced by pretreating patients with androgen deprivation. Neoadjuvant hormone therapy (NHT) was first reported in the 1940s. Renewed interest in NHT occurred with the advent of reversible forms of hormonal therapy. The optimal agent(s) and duration of therapy for NHT have yet to be determined. Sullivan found that serum PSA decreased to

TABLE 9.2. Results of Neoadjuvant Hormonal Therapy and Radical Prostatectomy for T3N0M0 Prostate Cancer

Author	*Number of Patients*	*Duration of Therapy (months)*	*pT2 Rate (%)*	*Mean PSA Preop*	*Mean Nadir PSA*
Andros[32]	16	4	19	39.1	0.43
Voges[64]	70	3	14.1	31.3	1.4
Schulmann[61]	15	3	27	—	—
Narayan[29]	30	3–10	14	204	4.3
Kennedy[65]	7	3–5	29	32.4	1.9

undetectable levels in 27% of patients after 3 months compared to 88% at 6 months.[60] A number of different agents and combinations have been used including antiandrogens, luteinizing hormone–releasing hormone (LH-RH) agonists, and 5-α-reductase inhibitors. No significant increase or decrease in surgical complications has been documented when prostatectomy is performed following NHT. Histologic interpretation of surgical specimens can be challenging in patients treated with NHT as special stains are often required to demonstrate residual tumor cells.

Attempts to decrease the incidence of microscopic T3 disease in men with clinically localized prostate cancer have shown some promise. Schulman noted a reduction in positive surgical margins from 57% to 32% when he compared patients undergoing surgery only to those who received NHT.[61] Labrie treated clinical T1 and T2 patients with NHT and found a reduction in pT3 disease from 29% to 13%.[62] Though NHT seems to decrease the number of patients found to have pT3 disease, long-term data regarding PSA recurrence and longevity are not yet available. It will be important to assess long-term efficacy of this therapy as it is unknown whether pT2 status after NHT portends the same prognosis as pT2 status following radical prostatectomy alone. A summary of the recent series comparing neoadjuvant hormonal therapy followed by radical prostatectomy with radical prostatectomy alone is displayed in Table 9.2.

Clinical T3 Disease

The utility of NHT in bulky T3 disease has generally not proved beneficial in rendering these patients disease-free postoperatively. One optimistic experience was reported by Labrie et al. who used 3 months of NHT with an antiandrogen and an LH-RH agonist in a small group (n = 15) of patients with T3 disease.[5] Positive margins in the control group were significantly more common (80%) than in the NHT group (14%). Despite Labrie's findings, the majority of series have demonstrated marginal or no benefit following NHT for stage C tumor. Plummer et al. treated patients with 4 months of either antiandrogen alone or antiandrogen plus an LH-RH agonist, and all but one patient had pathologic T3 disease.[63] Voges and colleagues used 3 months of combination NHT in 64 men prior to prostatectomy for T3 disease. Pathologic stages B, C, and D were found in 14%, 53%, and 33% respectively.[64] These percentages do not differ from series in which NHT was not given. Andros and colleagues treated 16 patients with 4 months of an antiandrogen and LH-RH agonist and only three of the surgical specimens had organ-confined disease.[32] Narayan et al. treated 30 men with stage C tumors for 3 to 10 months using a variety of hormonal therapies.[29] Forty-seven percent of patients were felt to be clinically downstaged to B disease after NHT, however, pathologic staging revealed only three patients (10%) to have organ-confined disease. The incidence of organ-confined disease in these studies is not better than the 4% to 30% clinical overstaging error of T3 tumors.[6–9] An ongoing phase II SWOG protocol (9109) is evaluating NHT using goserelin and flutamide in nonbulky stage C carcinoma of the prostate.

Neoadjuvant hormone therapy results in a 30% to 50% reduction in prostate size, and PSA values decrease by 95% to 99%. Unfortunately, the amount of gland size reduction and PSA level after NHT are not predictive of clinical or pathologic response. Among 64 patients with T3 disease treated with NHT, five men with nodal metastases and seven others with seminal vesicle invasion had a PSA less than 0.5 ng/ml after androgen deprivation.[64] The amount of PSA reduction is insignificant with respect to pathologic downstaging. Conversely, a poor response to NHT may be predictive since Schulman found that all patients with a PSA greater than 4.0 ng/ml after NHT had pT3 or pT4 disease.[61] Though histologic interpretation of prostatectomy specimens can be difficult after NHT, Kennedy found no change in Gleason scores attributable to NHT.[65] The literature regarding NHT is as yet inconclusive, though it appears that there is little chance of rendering patients with T3 disease tumor-free. The obvious downsizing of the prostate has not resulted in downstaging.

Radiation Therapy

Neoadjuvant hormone therapy prior to external beam radiation may have a potential role in the management of T3 prostate cancer. Radiation therapy depends on size or volume of disease for success, thus from a theoretic viewpoint, NHT should improve results. RTOG 8610 was begun in 1987 as an attempt to improve the percentage stem cell kill at the primary tumor site by reducing the number of stem cells necessary for radiotherapy to inactivate.[66] Maximum androgen blockade is accomplished using goserelin and flutamide for 2 months prior to XRT and for 2 months during radiation, and this was compared to XRT alone in the two study arms. After randomizing 45 patients with advanced local disease (unknown nodal status) and a follow-up of 3 years, the investigators report a clear advantage in patients treated with NHT. Local control in the NHT group was 84% versus 71% in the XRT only cohort. Disease-free survival (using PSA < 4.0 ng/ml as acceptable) was higher in the NHT group, 46% compared to 26%. This study is promising, though the short follow-up does not allow for evaluation of survival benefit.

CONCLUSIONS

Survival statistics for radical prostatectomy and external beam radiotherapy treatment of T3 carcinoma of the prostate are similar. Though neither is effective in curing T3 disease, prostatectomy is probably a better choice for the patient with significant local symptoms. At this time, neoadjuvant hormone therapy prior to radical prostatectomy has not been shown to downstage patients. Neoadjuvant hormone therapy prior to XRT may prove beneficial, though longer follow-up is mandatory. Patients with high-grade T3 disease will most likely derive no long-term benefit from any treatment modality. Young patients with low-grade disease should be offered curative treatment, while older patients with low-grade disease should be considered for expectant management. It is very important that well-developed clinical trials such as SWOG 8794, SWOG 9109, and RTOG 8610 are supported and completed, so that we may better determine the optimal management of the patient with stage T3 carcinoma of the prostate.

REFERENCES

1. Schmidt JD, Mettlin CJ, Natarajan N, et al: Trends in patient care for prostate cancer, 1974–1983: results of surveys by the American College of Surgeons. *J Urol* 136:416–421, 1986.
2. Mettlin CJ, Murphy GP: Prostate cancer. In Steele GD, Osteen RT, Winchester DP, et al: *National Cancer Data Base. Annual Review of Patient Care. 1994*. Atlanta, American Cancer Society, 1994, pp 87–96.
3. Mettlin C, Murphy GP, Lee F, et al: Characteristics of prostate cancer detected in the American Cancer Society–National Prostate Cancer Detection project. *J Urol* 152:1737–1740, 1994.
4. Fallon B, Williams RD: Current options in the management of clinical stage C prostate carcinoma. *Urol Clin North Am* 17:853–866, 1990.
5. Labrie F, Cusan L, Gomez J, et al: Downstaging of early stage prostate cancer before radical prostatectomy: the first randomized trial of neoadjuvant combination therapy with flutamide and LH-RH agonists. *Urology* 44:29–37, 1994.
6. Van den Ouden D, Davidson PJ, Hop W, et al: Radical prostatectomy as a monotherapy for locally advanced (stage T3) prostate cancer. *J Urol* 151:646–651, 1994.
7. Morgan WR, Bergstralh EJ, Zincke H: Long term evaluation of radical prostatectomy as treatment for clinical stage C (T3) prostate cancer. *Urology* 41:113–120, 1993.
8. Boxer RJ, Kaufman JJ, Goodwin WE: Radical prostatectomy for cancer of the prostate: 1951 to 1976. A review of 329 patients. *J Urol* 117:208–213, 1977.
9. Spaulding JT, Whitmore WF: Extended total excision of prostatic adenocarcinoma. *J Urol* 120:188–190, 1978.
10. Sands ME, Zagars GK, Pollack A, et al: Serum prostate-specific antigen, clinical stage, pathologic grade, and the incidence of nodal metastases in prostate cancer. *Urology* 44:215–220, 1994.
11. Greskovich FJ, Johnson DE, Tenney DM, et al: Prostate specific antigen in patients with clinical stage C prostate cancer: relation to lymph node status and grade. *J Urol* 145: 798–801, 1991.
12. Morgan WR, Zincke H: Radical retropubic prostatectomy as an alternative to definitive radiotherapy in selected patients with clinical stage C prostate cancer. *J Urol* 143:219A, 1990.
13. Rifkin HD, Zerhouni EA, Gatsonis CA, et al: Comparison of magnetic resonance imaging and ultrasonography in staging early prostate cancer. *N Engl J Med* 323:621–626, 1990.
14. Hricak H, Dooms GS, Jeffrey RB, et al: Prostate carcinoma: staging by clinical assessment, CT, and MR imaging. *Radiology* 162:331–336, 1987.
15. Chelsky MJ, Schnall MD, Seidmon EJ, et al: Use of endorectal surface coil magnetic resonance imaging for local staging of prostate cancer. *J Urol* 150:391–395, 1993.
16. Quinn SF, Franzini DA, Demlow TA, et al: MR imaging of prostate cancer with an endorectal surface coil technique: correlation with whole mount specimens. *Radiology* 190: 323–327, 1994.

17. Cummings JM, Boullier JA, Sankari BR, et al: Seminal vesicle volume as a sonographic predictor of prostate cancer stage. *Urology* 44:206–210, 1994.

18. Lowe FC, Trauzzi SJ: Prostatic acid phosphatase in 1993. Its limited clinical utility. *Urol Clin North Am* 20:589–595, 1993.

19. Burnett AL, Chan DW, Brendler CB, et al: The value of serum enzymatic acid phosphatase in the staging of localized prostate cancer. *J Urol* 148:1832–1834, 1992.

20. Kucuk O, Demirer T, Gilman-Sachs A, et al: Intratumor heterogeneity of DNA ploidy and correlations with clinical stage and histologic grade in prostate cancer. *J Surg Oncol* 54:171–174, 1993.

21. Stege R, Lundh B, Tribukait B, et al: Deoxyribonucleic acid ploidy and the direct assay of prostatic acid phosphatase and prostate specific antigen in fine needle aspiration biopsies as diagnostic methods in prostate cancer. *J Urol* 144:299–302, 1990.

22. Schellhammer PF: Radical prostatectomy. Patterns of local failure and survival in 67 patients. *Urology* 31:191–197, 1988.

23. Epstein JI, Carmichael MJ, Pizov G, et al: Influence of capsular penetration on progression following radical prostatectomy: a study of 196 cases with long term followup. *J Urol* 150:135–141, 1993.

24. Valiancien G, Bochereau G, Wetzel O, et al: Influence of preoperative positive seminal vesicle biopsy in the staging of prostate cancer. *J Urol* 152:1152–1156, 1994.

25. Zagars GK, von Eschenbach AC, Johnson DE, et al: Stage C adenocarcinoma of the prostate. An analysis of 551 patients treated with external beam radiation. *Cancer* 60:1489–1499, 1987.

26. Babian RJ, Zagars GK, Ayala AG: Radiation therapy of stage C prostate cancer: significance of Gleason grade to survival. *Semin Urol* 4:225–231, 1990.

27. Wilson LD, Ennis R, Percarpio B, et al: Location of the prostatic apex and its relationship to the ischial tuberosities. *Int J Radiat Oncol Biol Phys* 29:1133–1138, 1994.

28. Schellhammer PF, El-Mahdi AM, Kuban DA: Local failure and related complications after definitive treatment of clinical stage C cancer of the prostate by irradiation or surgery. *Semin Urol* 4:232–246, 1990.

29. Narayan P, Lowe BA, Carroll PR, et al: Neoadjuvant hormonal therapy and radical prostatectomy for clinical stage C carcinoma of the prostate. *Br J Urol* 73:544–548, 1994.

30. Zagars GK, Geara FB, Pollack A, et al: The T classification of clinically localized prostate cancer. An appraisal based on disease outcome after radiation therapy. *Cancer* 73: 1904–1912, 1994.

31. Corn BW, Hanks GE, Lee WR, et al: Do the current subclassifications of stage T3 adenocarcinoma of the prostate have clinical relevance? *Urology* 45:484–490, 1995.

32. Andros EA, Danesghari F, Crawford ED: Neoadjuvant hormonal therapy in stage C adenocarcinoma of the prostate. *Clin Invest Med* 16:510–515, 1993.

33. Kabalin JN, Hodge KK, McNeal JE, et al: Identification of residual cancer in prostate following radiation therapy: role of transrectal ultrasound guided biopsy and prostate specific antigen. *J Urol* 142:326–331, 1989.

34. See WA, Williams WD: Management of prostate cancer. Stage by stage. In Das S, Crawford ED: *Cancer of the Prostate*. New York, Marcel Dekker, 1993, p 408.

35. Zagars GK, von Eschenbach AC, Ayala AG, et al: The influence of local control on metastatic dissemination of prostate cancer treated by external beam megavoltage radiation therapy. *Cancer* 68:2370–2377, 1991.

36. Kaplan ID, Prestidge BR, Bagshaw MA, et al: The importance of local control in the treatment of prostate cancer. *J Urol* 147:917–921, 1992.

37. Thompson IM: Clinical stage C carcinoma of the prostate. *AUA Update Series* 11:82–87, 1993.
38. Holzman M, Carlton CE, Scardino PT: The frequency and morbidity of local tumor recurrence after definitive radiotherapy for stage C prostate cancer. *J Urol* 146:1578–1582, 1991.
39. Kahn K, Thompson W, Bush S, et al: Transperineal percutaneous Iridium-192 interstitial template implantation of the prostate: results and complications in 321 patients. *Int J Radiat Oncol Biol Phys* 22:935–939, 1992.
40. Moul JW, Paulson DF: The role of radical surgery in the management of radiation recurrent and large volume prostate cancer. *Cancer* 68:1265–1271, 1991.
41. Gonder MH, Soanes WA, Smith V: Experimental prostate cryosurgery. *Invest Urol* 1:610–618, 1964.
42. Flocks RH, O'Donoghue EPN, Milleman LA, et al: Management of stage C prostate carcinoma. *Urol Clin North Am* 2:163–179, 1975.
43. Bonney WW, Fallon B, Gerber W: Cryosurgery in prostatic cancer: survival. *Urology* 19:37–42, 1982.
44. Loening S, Lubaroff D: Cryosurgery and immunotherapy for prostate cancer. *Urol Clin North Am* 11:327–336, 1984.
45. Littrup PJ, Montie J, Mody A, et al: Prostate cryotherapy: ultrasonographic and pathologic correlation in the canine model. *Urology* 44:175–184, 1994.
46. Miller RJ, Cohen JK, Merlott LA: Percutaneous transperineal cryosurgical ablation of the prostate for the primary treatment of clinical stage C adenocarcinoma of the prostate. *Urology* 44:170–174, 1994.
47. Rozanski TA, Faerber GJ: Massive locally extensive prostate cancer. *Urology* 43:242–243, 1994.
48. Byar DP: The Veterans Administration Cooperative Urological Research Group's studies of cancer of the prostate. *Cancer* 32:1126–1130, 1973.
49. Blackard CE: Re: deferred treatment of low grade stage T3 prostate cancer without distant metastases (letter; comment). *J Urol* 151:436, 1994.
50. Crawford ED, Eisenberger MA, McLeod DG, et al: A controlled trial of leuprolide with and without flutamide in prostatic carcinoma. *N Engl J Med* 321:419–424, 1989.
51. Fleshner NE, Trachtenberg J: Treatment of advanced prostate cancer with the combination of finasteride plus flutamide: early results. *Eur Urol* (suppl)2:106–112, 1993.
52. Adolfsson J: Deferred treatment of low grade stage T3 prostate cancer without distant metastases. *J Urol* 149:326–328, 1993.
53. Hanno PM: Carcinoma of the prostate—stage C. In Seidmon EJ, Hanno PM: *Current Urologic Therapy*, ed 3. Philadelphia, Saunders, 1994, p 384.
54. Aro J, Haapiainen R, Kajanti M, et al: Comparison of endocrine and radiation therapy in locally advanced prostatic cancer. *Eur Urol* 15:182–186, 1988.
55. Carter GE, Lieskovsky G, Skinner DG, et al: Results of local and/or systemic adjuvant therapy in the management of pathological stage C or D1 prostate cancer following radical prostatectomy. *J Urol* 142:1266–1271, 1989.
56. Schild SE, Wong WW, Grado GL, et al: Radiotherapy for isolated increases in serum prostate-specific antigen levels after radical prostatectomy. *Mayo Clin Proc* 69:613–619, 1994.
57. McCarthy JF, Catalona WJ, Hudson MA: Effect of radiation therapy on detectable serum prostate specific antigen levels following radical prostatectomy: early versus delayed treatment. *J Urol* 151:1575–1578, 1994.

58. Thompson IM, Paradelo JC, Crawford ED, et al: An opportunity to determine optimal treatment of pT3 prostate cancer: the window may be closing. *Urology* 44:804–811, 1994.

59. Cheng WS, Frydenberg M, Bergstralh EJ, et al: Radical prostatectomy for pathologic stage C prostate cancer: influence of pathologic variables and adjuvant treatment on disease outcome. *Urology* 42:283–291, 1993.

60. Sullivan L, Gleave M, Goldenberg L, et al: Long term neoadjuvant hormonal therapy prior to radical prostatectomy in localized prostate cancer. *J Urol* 151:435A, 1994.

61. Schulman CC: Neoadjuvant androgen blockade prior to prostatectomy: a retrospective study and critical review. *Prostate Suppl* 5:9–14, 1994.

62. Labrie F, Dupont A, Gomez JL, et al: Beneficial effect of combination therapy administered prior to radical prostatectomy. *J Urol* 149:348A, 1994.

63. Plummer K, Crawford ED, Daneshgari F, et al: Hormonal pretreatment does not affect the final pathologic stage of locally advanced prostate cancer. *Urology* 44:38–42, 1994.

64. Voges GE, Mottrie AM, Stockle M, et al: Hormone therapy prior to radical prostatectomy in patients with clinical stage C prostate cancer. *Prostate Suppl* 5:4–8, 1994.

65. Kennedy TJ, Sonneland AM, Marlett MM, et al: Luteinizing hormone–releasing hormone downstaging of clinical stage C prostate cancer. *J Urol* 147:891–893, 1992.

66. Shipley WU: Radiation Therapy Oncology Group: Phase III trial of androgen suppression before and during radiation therapy for locally advanced prostatic cancer: abstract report of RTOG 8610. *Prostate Suppl* 5:2–3, 1994.

10

Treatment of Stage D2 Prostate Cancer

Robert C. Flanigan
Sean P. Manion

Adenocarcinoma of the prostate is the most common cancer among American men with approximately 200,000 cases diagnosed annually and 38,000 deaths attributed to this disease.[1] This accounts for approximately 10% of all cancer deaths in men. Metastatic disease is diagnosed in over one-third of patients found to have prostate cancer.[2] Eighty-five percent of patients with stage D1 prostate cancer (node positive) progress to distant metastasis (stage D2 disease) within 5 years and those with stage D2 disease display a median survival of approximately 2½ years.[3] In this chapter we will discuss the various treatment options for advanced prostate cancer as well as the scientific basis for these treatments.

ANDROGEN REGULATION

The primary work of Huggins and Hodges in 1941 established the basis of hormonal manipulation for treatment of prostate cancer. This landmark study demonstrated the effectiveness of castration which has been the cornerstone of treatment for metastatic disease over the past five decades.[4] Sixty to 80% of patients with prostate cancer will demonstrate subjective and objective responses to castration including a decrease in primary and metastatic tumor burden, relief of bladder outlet and ureteral obstruction, and improvement in bone pain.[5]

Androgen production is under the regulation of pituitary hormones (Fig. 10.1). Luteinizing hormone–releasing hormone (LH-RH) is released from the hypothalamus stimulating luteinizing hormone (LH) production and release from the anterior pituitary. LH in turn stimulates testicular Leydig cell secretion of androgens. Testosterone circulates in the plasma bound to albumin and testosterone–estradiol binding globulin. Only approximately 2% of testosterone is free in serum and is available to diffuse into the

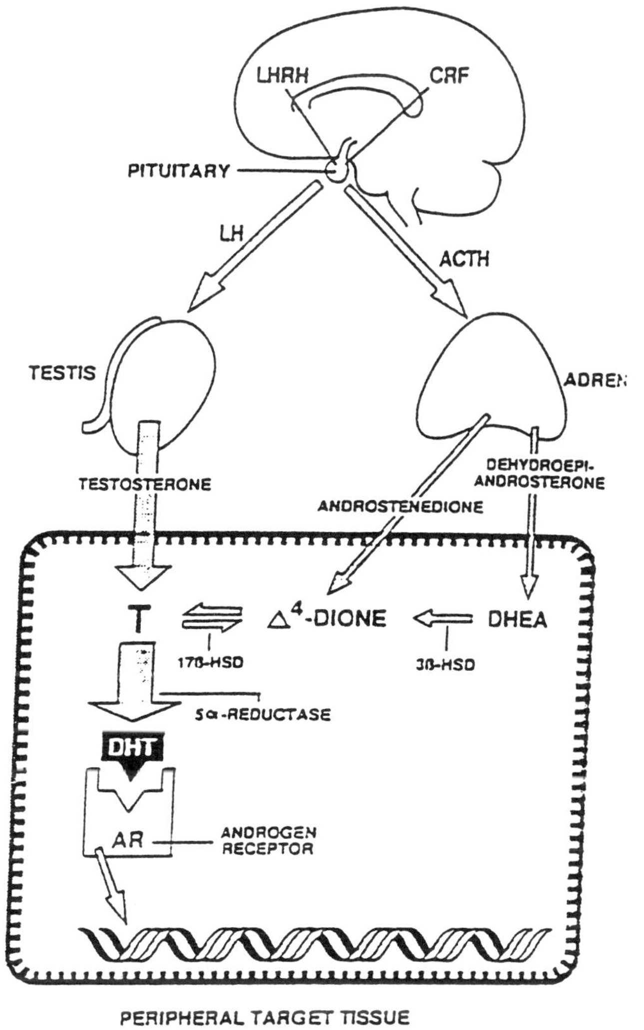

Fig. 10.1. Intracrine activity of the human prostate or biosynthetic steps involved in the formation of the active androgen DHT from testicular testosterone and from the adrenal precursors DHEA and Δ^4-dione in human prostatic tissue. 17ß-HSD = 17ß-hydroxysteroid dehydrogenase; 3ß-HSD = 3ß-hydroxysteroid dehydrogenase/Δ5-Δ4-isomerase. The width of the arrows indicates the relative importance of the testis (60%) and adrenal gland (40%) as sources of DHT. The testis secretes testosterone (T), which is transformed in most peripheral tissues into the more potent androgen DHT. This in turn, interacts with the androgen receptor and activates the expression of genes mediating androgen-specific functions, including cell growth. Instead of secreting T or DHT directly, the adrenal secretes large amounts of DHEA, DHEA S, and Δ^4 dione, which are transported in the blood to the peripheral tissues. These sites transform these inactive precursors into the active androgens T and DHT. The enzymatic complexes 3ß HSD, 17ß-HSD, and 5-α-reductase required for the transformation of DHEA and Δ^4-dione into T and DHT are present in the prostatic cells, thus making possible adjustments in the supply of androgens. The testis possesses the five enzymes, namely, cholesterol side-chain cleavage (P-450scc), 17α-hydroxylase desmolase (P45017α), 3ß-HSD, 17ß-HSD, and 5-α-reductase, which permit the formation of DHT from cholesterol. However, many peripheral tissues, including the prostate, possess 17ß HSD, 3ß HSD, and 5-α-reductase, which are sufficient to convert adrenal DHEA or Δ^4-dione into T and DHT for local use. From Labrie F, Belanger A, Simard J et al. Combined therapy for Prostate Cancer. Endocrine & biologic basis of its choice as new standard first-line therapy. *Cancer (Suppl)* 71:1059, 1993. Reproduced with permission.

prostate cell. Testosterone mainly acts as a prohormone undergoing enzymatic conversion to dihydrotestosterone by 5-α-reductase or is aromatized to estrogens in the peripheral tissue for subsequent hormonal-mediated action.

The negative feedback of androgens and estrogens occurs at both the hypothalamic and pituitary level.[6] This hypothalamic pituitary–gonadal axis accounts for approximately 95% of circulating testosterone. The remaining circulating testosterone is produced by the zona reticularis of the adrenal gland. Hypothalamic release of corticotropin-releasing hormone (CRH) stimulates release of adrenocorticotropic hormone (ACTH) which in turn stimulates adrenal production and release of androgens. Negative feedback of adrenal steroids occurs at the hypothalamic and pituitary level.

TESTOSTERONE'S EFFECT ON PROSTATE TISSUE

Within the prostate tissue, testosterone and adrenal androgens are converted to dihydrotestosterone via the 5-α-reductase enzyme. Both testosterone and dihydrotestosterone combine with intracellular protein receptors and this hormone–receptor complex facilitates DNA transcription within the cell nucleus. This androgen-mediated transcription is essential to cellular homeostasis in regulation of tissue growth. The conversion of testosterone to dihydrotestosterone confirms a specificity which accounts for a several fold greater affinity of this complex for dihydrotestosterone over testosterone.

PROGNOSTIC FACTORS

Androgen deprivation therapy continues to be the treatment of choice for patients with metastatic adenocarcinoma of the prostate. Although no single factor is able to predict tumor response to androgen deprivation, many clinical, radiographic, and laboratory variables have been assessed with respect to their ability to predict response to treatment and patient prognosis. These prognostic factors allow the clinician to determine treatment modalities, adjust treatment intensity, and counsel patients appropriately. Grade and stage of tumor at initial diagnosis has proven to be a significant prognostic factor, although its usefulness in metastatic disease is less certain.[7] Studies comparing a patient's age with outcomes have demonstrated that those patients less than 60 years of age or greater than 80 years of age have a significantly poorer prognosis compared to those between the ages of 60–80.[8] Patients with fewer than six metastatic lesions on bone scans have also demonstrated a significantly better 2-year survival than those with more extensive disease. Improved prognosis has been demonstrated in patients with decreased bone pain, nominal analgesic use, and improved performance status.[7] However, most patients with metastatic prostate cancer begin treatment prior to decline in performance status, thus limiting the clinical utility of this parameter. Laboratory variables including elevated alkaline phosphatase, hemoglobin less than 12 gm/day and below normal pretreatment serum testosterone levels have also proven to be poor prognostic variables.[9] Many studies have demonstrated pretreatment prostatic specific antigen (PSA) levels to be inversely proportional to survival with an elevated PSA associated with a greater likelihood of tumor recurrence and a shorter time to progression.[10] Conversely, normalization of PSA after treatment or a decline in PSA by greater than 90% is associated with prolonged progression-free survival.

TREATMENT MODALITIES

Over the years, medical technology has dramatically improved our ability to alter the hormonal milieu, affecting both androgen production and recognition. This has created a plethora of options available to effect the growth of prostate cancer through hormonal regulation and androgen deprivation (Table 10.1).

Surgical castration is the oldest and most assured method to eliminate Leydig cell testosterone production. Surgical castration removes approximately 95% of circulating androgens. The procedure has few complications; is immediate, permanent, and ensures total patient compliance. One of the major criticisms of surgical castration is the psychological effects this procedure poses to many men.

Medical castration can be reliably achieved by oral estrogen administration.[11] Estrogens act by suppressing pituitary luteinizing hormone release by competitive inhibition, increasing hepatic production of testosterone–estrogen binding globulin (thus, decreasing the amount of free testosterone), and interfering with testosterone binding. The most common oral estrogen available is diethylstilbestrol (DES). The original data from the Veterans Administration Cooperative Urology Group (VACUG) demonstrated DES 5 mg

TABLE 10.1. Current First Line Hormonal Treatments Used in Metastatic Prostate Cancer

Surgical castration
Bilateral orchiectomy
Subcapsular orchiectomy
Subepididymal orchiectomy
Medial castration
Estrogens
Diethylstilbestrol 1–3 mg/day
Luteinizing hormone–releasing hormone agonists/antagonists
Luprolide
Buserelin
Goserelin
Nafarelin
Pure nonsteroidal antiandrogens
Flutamide
Nilutamide
Casodex
Steroidal antiandrogens
Megestrol acetate
Cyproterone acetate
Adrenal suppression
Ketoconazole
Spironolactone
Aminoglutethimide

per day to be as effective as surgical castration. However, cardiovascular complications at this dose were significant and lower doses have since been evaluated. DES at 3 mg and 1 mg have both been evaluated and been proven to reliably reduce serum testosterone to the castrate range while decreasing cardiovascular side effects.[12] Unfortunately, even at a dosage range of 3 mg/day, cardiovascular complications are nearly 3 times that of patients not treated with oral estrogens.[13]

Luteinizing hormone–releasing hormone analogs (LH-RH-A) were initially developed for the treatment of infertility and were found to promote pituitary luteinizing hormone secretion. After an initial rise in luteinizing hormone and testosterone production lasting 7–10 days, luteinizing hormone and testosterone are suppressed secondary to downregulation of luteinizing hormone–releasing hormone receptors and postreceptor events. This results in a decreased plasma testosterone level to the castrate range.[14] This effect persists for the duration of treatment with LH-RH-A and is completely reversible after treatment is discontinued. Common side effects with LH-RH-A include impotence (84%), hot flashes (63%), and breast swelling (5%).[15] In addition, approximately 5% of patients undergoing LH-RH analog treatment suffer clinically apparent "flare phenomenon" due to the initial LH surge. The "flare phenomena" can be minimized by the concominant use of androgen receptor blockers or DES. Various luteinizing hormone–releasing hormone analogs have been developed including lupride, goserelin, buserelin, and nafarelin which are generally administered as depot injections on a monthly basis (3-month depot preparations are currently being evaluated).

Pure nonsteroidal antiandrogens block the intracellular androgen receptor for testosterone and dihydrotestosterone. The three current nonsteroidal antiandrogens, flutamide, nilutamide, and casodex are structurally similar. Although current research is underway evaluating antiandrogens as primary monotherapy, their current use is in combination with medical or surgical castration for total androgen blockade or as a means for effectively blocking luteinizing hormone surge or "flare phenomenon." When used as monotherapy, one of the important benefits of these agents is the preservation of potency in the majority of patients. Adverse effects include elevated serum testosterone produced by receptor blockade of the hypothalamic and pituitary androgen receptors resulting in increased LH production and subsequent increased testosterone production.[16] Gynecomastia (produced by the unopposed estrogen effect on breast tissue), gastrointestinal disturbances (particularly diarrhea), and liver toxicity also may limit their use.

Steroidal antiandrogens offer a combined mode of androgen suppressions by blocking the intracellular androgen receptor and inhibiting 5-α-reductase, while, in addition, inhibiting luteinizing hormone release from the pituitary due to their progestational component.[16] Megestrol acetate and cyproterone acetate are the most commonly used steroidal antiandrogens. Studies comparing cyproterone acetate to diethylstilbestrol at a dose of 3 mg per day have demonstrated equal efficacy with a decrease in the cardiovascular side effects in the cyproterone acetate group.[17] Steroidal antiandrogen treatment indications include monotherapy, combined therapy with medical or surgical castration for total androgen ablation, and the prevention of "flare phenomenon" during LH-RH analog administration. It is essential that steroid antiandrogens be coadministered with estrogen such as DES in a dose of 0.1 mg/day to prevent the effects of the escape phenomena which occur after several months of monotherapy.[18]

Clinical studies by Huggins in the 1940s demonstrated the effect of bilateral adrenalectomy in the treatment of refractory prostate cancer.[19] Numerous drugs are presently available which accomplish medical adrenalectomy. The three most common drugs in this group are ketoconazole, spironolactone, and aminoglutethimide. Ketoconazole is an antimycotic agent which blocks both testosterone and adrenal steroidal production by interfering with the cytochrome P450 complex.[20] Spironolactone inhibits the enzymes 17-α-hydroxylase and 17, 20-desmolase, effectively halting adrenal and gonadal steroidal production.[16] Aminoglutethimide, initially introduced as an anticonvulsant, blocks the 20, 24-desmolase enzyme system, thus inhibiting the conversion of cholesterol to pregnenolone.[16] Prolonged use of these medications requires mineral corticoid and glucocorticoid replacement.[21] Some authors have suggested that it is the steroid replacement and not the adrenal androgen production blockade which is responsible for the moderate clinical benefit demonstrated by the use of these agents.[22]

TOTAL ANDROGEN BLOCKADE

Although most patients with metastatic prostate cancer respond initially to androgen deprivation therapy, 20–40% will not respond to hormonal treatment while those who do respond will fail over time.[5] This lack of response and failure over time is believed to result from development of androgen-independent prostate cancer. The cause of this independence appears to be heterogeneity within the prostate cancer cell population. The development of this heterogeneous population is speculative and controversial. Two theories have been postulated to explain the development of hormonal independence seen in prostate cancer.[23] The first theory, known as the environmental selection model, assumes that the initial prostate cancer is heterogeneous with respect to androgen requirements. Thus, the tumor is composed of androgen-dependent as well as androgen-independent cells from its inception. In this model, androgen deprivation affects only the androgen-dependent cells, allowing the androgen-independent cell lines to continue to grow in a noncompetitive environment. An alternative theory, known as the environmental adaption model, presumes that the prostate cancer is initially homogeneous with respect to the requirement of androgen to stimulate growth. Following androgen ablation, these androgen-dependent cells undergo environmental pressure to become androgen-independent. It is speculated that the introduction of antiandrogens might delay the development of the androgen-insensitive cell lines, thus inhibiting prostate cancer growth. It is this theory that forms the basis for total androgen deprivation.

The concept of total androgen blockade was first introduced in 1945 by the work of Huggins and Scott. They performed bilateral adrenalectomies with the intention of total androgen deprivation. The rationale for complete androgen deprivation is based in the finding that although the level of circulating androgens is reduced 90–95% after orchiectomy or hormonal therapy, the concentration of dihydrotestosterone in the prostate tissue is merely reduced to 60–75%. This remaining 25–40% of prostatic androgens are available to promote the growth of androgen-dependent prostate cancer.[24] The source of the remaining androgens is the adrenal gland and it is the blockade of these adrenally produced androgens in combination with medical or surgical castration which forms the basis of total androgen deprivation.

Several prospective, randomized trials have been performed to evaluate theoretical benefits of total androgen suppression. The Canadian trial compared orchiectomy + placebo to orchiectomy + nilutamide. A total of 208 patients were compared to evaluate efficacy of this therapy. Although there was an increase in median survival of 5.4 months with respect to the orchiectomy + nilutamide group, there was no statistically significant difference between the two groups with respect to progression or survival.[25] The European Organization of Research and Treatment of Cancer (EORTC) compared orchiectomy versus goserelin + flutamide in a trial composed of 327 men with prostate cancer. Preliminary results did not demonstrate any survival advantage with the combination treatment. However, analysis of the mature data demonstrated a significant difference in favor of the combination treatment group with respect to time to objective progression, subjective progression, time to first progression, and duration of survival, with a median duration of survival of 27.1 months versus 34.4 months in favor of the total androgen suppression group. In particular, comparing duration of survival based on death due to malignant disease, there was a statistically significant difference with a median time to death of 28.8 versus 43.9 months.[26]

To date, the strongest study supporting the benefit of total androgen suppression was performed by the National Cancer Institute (NCI).[27] In this study, lupron was compared to lupron versus flutamide in 603 patients with stage D2 prostate cancer. This placebo-controlled, randomized double-blind study demonstrated a statistically significant difference to progression (16.5 months versus 13.5 months) and survival (35.6 months versus 28 months); all deaths ~ 8 months. Further evaluation demonstrated patients with minimal disease and good performance status obtained the greatest benefits from combination therapy with an increase in survival of almost 2 years (Fig. 10.2).[28] Additional studies comparing various means of total androgen ablation are presently underway in North

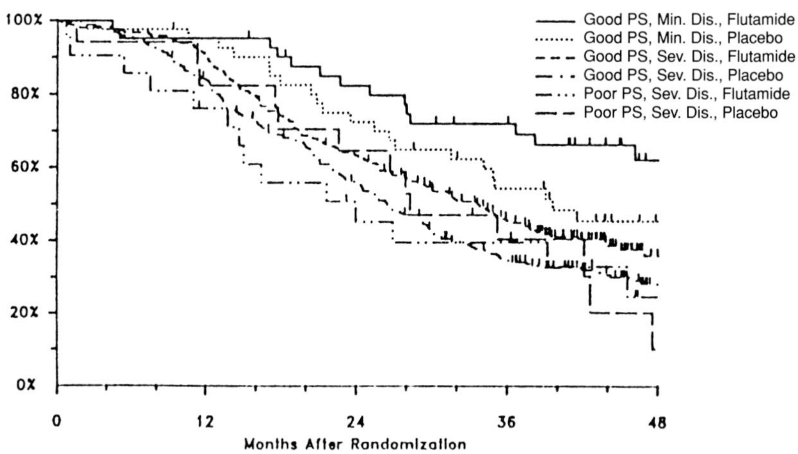

	AT RISK	EVENTS	MEDIAN IN MONTHS
Good PS, Min. Dis., Flutamide	41	15	51.9
Good PS, Min. Dis., Placebo	41	22	39.6
Good PS, Sev. Dis., Flutamide	241	144	33.6
Good PS, Sev. Dis., Placebo	241	164	26.4
Poor PS, Sev. Dis., Flutamide	21	14	23.9
Poor PS, Sev. Dis., Placebo	17	13	28.3

Fig. 10.2. National Cancer Institute Intergroup Protocol 003G: Survival classified by stratification and randomized treatment. December 1989. From Crawford ED, Blumenstein BA, Goodman PJ et al. Leuprolide with and without flutamide in advanced prostate cancer. *Cancer (Suppl)* 66:1039, 1990. Reproduced with permission.

America and Europe including the Intergroup NCI trial of orchiectomy + placebo versus orchiectomy + flutamide which has just completed accrual.

PATIENTS WITH ANDROGEN INSENSITIVITY

Standard treatment for metastatic prostate cancer has been androgen deprivation therapy due to its proven efficacy (greater than 80% response) and minimal side effects. Unfortunately, of those that do respond, the majority will relapse in 18–24 months after the initiation of hormonal therapy. Secondary hormonal therapy after initial hormonal failure utilizing high-dose estrogens, antiandrogens, or androgen synthesis inhibitors has been disappointing. Subjective results can occur in 10–20% of patients with a duration of approximately 6 months.[29]

CHEMOTHERAPY

Although a small number of trials have evaluated chemotherapy in newly diagnosed D2 prostate cancer, chemotherapy has traditionally been preserved for hormonal failure patients and, in general, results have been disappointing. The poor response rates of metastatic prostate cancer to chemotherapy are due to both tumor and patient factors.

In general, most therapeutic trials have been limited to patients with end-stage disease who have large tumor burdens. There is a known inverse relationship between tumor size and curability with large tumors having a substantial number of cells in a nonproliferative state and large tumor burden inhibiting the ability of chemotherapeutic agents to properly penetrate the mass so as to achieve adequate tissue levels. Chemotherapeutic agents are toxic to dividing cells and those tumors with a high growth fractions are most often susceptible. Prostate cancer, however, has an extremely long doubling time (in some cases greater than one year) with a low mitotic index which likely plays a major role in its relative chemotherapeutic resistance.

In a review of 26 drug trials, Yagoda and Petrylak demonstrated objective response to chemotherapeutic agents in only 8.7% of patients with only six agents having an objective response of greater than 10%.[30] This report confirmed earlier reports that hormonally resistant adenocarcinoma of the prostate fails to respond to most cytotoxic chemotherapeutic agents. The most notable of those agents having an objective response of greater than 10% include vinblastine with a partial response of 21%,[31] trimetrexate with a partial response of 17%,[32] and estramustine with a partial response of 14%.[33] However, in all cases responses were short-lived. Combination chemotherapeutic agents have been tried, however, they have demonstrated similarly poor responses.[34] The combination of estramustine and vinblastine appears to be the most effective regimen to date. Objective responses (defined as decreased serum PSA level by ≥50%) were obtained in 30–50% of patients treated after hormonal failure.[35]

Immunotherapy protocols involving interferons have likewise revealed disappointing results. Recent studies involving prostate specific monoclonal antibodies linked to cytotoxic compounds represent a promising and innovative approach to the treatment of metastatic prostate cancer.

Suramin is a synthetic compound initially developed as an antiparacytic agent. The antineoplastic activity of suramin is based on its ability to affect the growth of prostate cancer via numerous mechanisms. Suramin binds to and disrupts the function of cell surface and intracellular enzymes, thus inhibiting multiple growth factor functions. Suramin also suppresses in vitro colony formation inhibition, and functions as an adrenocorticolytic agent. Objective responses lasting one year have occurred in approximately one-third of patients.[36] Modest success in clinical trials makes this agent one of the most promising for treatment of hormonal refractory prostate cancer. Toxicities are significant including hematologic and infectious complications as well as peripheral neuropathy.

PALLIATIVE RADIATION THERAPY

Radiation therapy has long been used as primary treatment of prostatic cancer localized to the prostate. The role of radiation therapy in metastatic prostate cancer centers on palliation of symptomatic bone pain. Patients with metastatic prostate cancer frequently develop multiple focal areas of bone pain which occur simultaneously and are refractory to opioid analgesics. One rational approach to this dilemma is the treatment modality involving hemibody radiation (Fig. 10.3). Using this technique, the body is divided into upper and lower fields at the level of the umbilicus. Doses of 400–1,000 cGy have produced complete pain relief in 24–70% of patients undergoing this treatment with partial relief in 24–71%.[37] The relief occurs within 24 hr in the majority of patients. After 4–6 weeks, the opposite field can be irradiated allowing for blood cell levels to return to baseline. This treatment does not appear to offer any significant prolongation in survival. Side effects include nausea, vomiting, fever, diarrhea, tachycardia, and hypotension; tend to be minor and in a majority of patients, resolve within 24 hr.

Strontium-89 is a β-emitting isotope which decays with a half-life of 50.5 days. It localizes to areas of increased mineral turnover within the body following the biologic pathways of calcium. Because of this selectivity, diseased bone receives approximately 10 times the irradiation of healthy marrow.[38] Following injection, pain relief typically occurs between 10–20 days with a main duration of 6 months.[39] Clinical trials in North America and Europe demonstrated strontium-89 to be as effective as hemibody radiation (70–80% pain relief) with fewer side effects. Major side effects encountered included thrombocytopenia and leukocytopenia, which are generally mild, dose-dependent, and reversible.

FLUTAMIDE WITHDRAWAL SYNDROME

Recent reports have demonstrated that patients treated with hormonal combinations including flutamide who progress to hormonal-insensitive prostate cancer demonstrate clinical improvement and objective decline in PSA values with the cessation of flutamide therapy lasting approximately 6 months.[40] The precise mechanism of this phenomenon has not been defined. Nonetheless, approximately 25–30% of patients so treated will, in our experience, demonstrate a decrease in PSA upon cessation of flutamide.

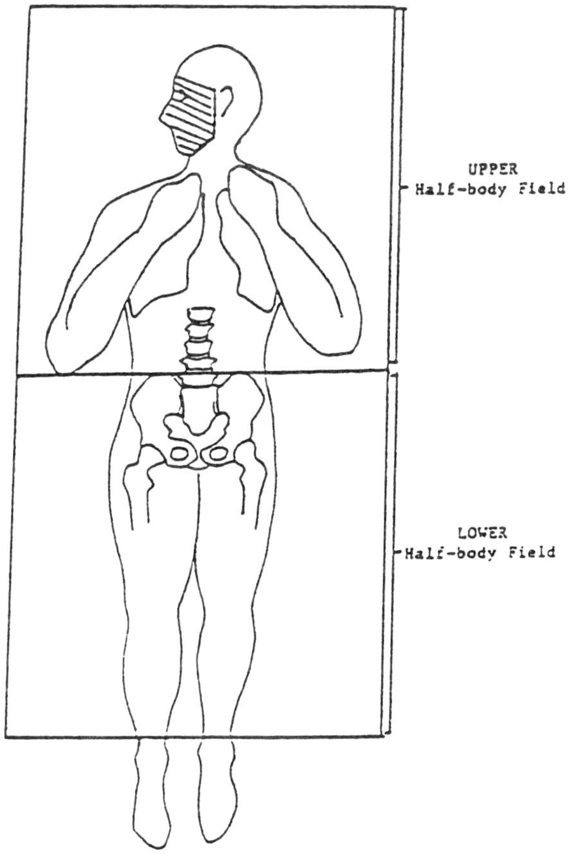

Fig. 10.3. Standard fields for half-body irradiation. From Kuban DA, Schellhammer PF, El-Mahdi AM. Hemibody irradiation in advanced prostatic carcinoma. *UCNA* 18:131, 1991. Reproduced with permission

SPINAL CORD COMPRESSION

When a patient with prostate cancer presents with symptomatic vertebral involvement, the patient should be treated with high-dose steroids. Those patients not previously treated with hormonal therapy may undergo complete androgen suppression via orchiectomy, ketoconazole, spironolactone, or aminoglutethimide because of the immediate actions of these therapies in reducing the level of serum testosterone. Radiation therapy also plays a critical role in the treatment of spinal cord compression. Surgical decompression of the cord is generally reserved for patients who have previously undergone radiation therapy and those with spinal instability.

REFERENCES

1. Boring CC, Squires T, Tong T: Cancer statistics 1994. *Cancer* 44:7, 1994.
2. Mettlin C, Jones GW, Murphy GP: Trends in prostate cancer care in the U.S., 1974–1990: ob-

servations from the patient care evaluation studies of the American College of Surgeons Commission on Cancer. *CA Cancer J Clin* 43:83–91, 1993.

3. Kozlowski JM, Grayhack JT: Carcinoma of the prostate. In Gillenwater JY, Grayhack JT, Howard SS, et al: *Adult and Pediatric Urology*, ed 2. Chicago, Year Book Medical Publishers, 1991.
4. Huggins C, Hodges CV: Studies on prostate cancer I: the effect of castration, of estrogen and of androgen injection of serum phosphates in metastatic carcinoma of the prostate. *Cancer Res* 1:293, 1941.
5. Resnick ML, Grayhack JT: Treatment of stage IV carcinoma of the prostate. *Urol Clin North Am* 2:141, 1975.
6. McCann SM: The anterior pituitary and hypothalamus. In Griffin JE, Ojeda SR: *Textbook of Endocrine Physiology*. New York, Oxford University Press, 1988.
7. deVoogt HJ, Suciu S, Sylvester R, et al: Prognostic factor analysis from EORTC trials in advanced prostate cancer. *Prog Clin Biol Res* 357:69–72, 1990.
8. Wilson JM, Kemp IW, Stein GJ: Cancer of the prostate. Do younger men have a poorer survival rate? *Br J Urol* 56:391–396, 1984.
9. Soloway MS, Oshikawa S, VanderZwaag R, et al: Prognostic factors in patients with advanced prostate cancer. *Urology* 33(suppl):53–56, 1989.
10. Matykin H, Perito PE, Soloway MS: Prognostic factors in metastatic prostate cancer. *Cancer* (Suppl) 72(12):3788–3791, 1993.
11. Citrin DL, Kies MS, Wallenmark CB, et al: A phase II study of high dose estrogens in prostate cancer. *Cancer* 56:457, 1985.
12. Veteran's Administration Cooperative Urologic Research Group: Carcinoma of the prostate: treatment comparisons. *J Urol* 98:516, 1967.
13. Byar DP: The Veteran's Administration Cooperative Urological Research Group's studies of cancer of the prostate: *Cancer* 32:1126, 1973.
14. Labrie F, Belanger A, Cusan L, et al: Antifertility effects of LHRH agonists in the male. *J Androl* 1:209, 1980.
15. Kaisary AV, Tyrrell CJ, Peeling WB, et al: Comparison of LHRH analog (Zoladex) with orchiectomy in patients with metastatic prostate carcinoma. *Br J Urol* 67:502, 1991.
16. Daneshgari F, Crawford DE: Endocrine therapy of advanced cancer of the prostate. *Cancer* (Suppl)71:1089, 1993.
17. Pavone-Macaluso M, deVoogt HJ, Viggiano G, et al: Comparison of DES, cyproterone acetate and medroxyprogesterone acetate in the treatment of advanced prostate cancer: final analysis of a randomized phase III trial of the European Organization for Research on Treatment of Cancer Urological Group. *J Urol* 136:624, 1986.
18. Geller J: Megestrol acetate plus low dose estrogens in the management of advanced prostate cancer. *Urol Clin North Am* 18:83, 1991.
19. Huggins C, Scott WW: Bilateral adrenalectomy in prostate cancer: clinical features and urinary excretion of 17-ketosteroids and estrogens. *Ann Surg* 122:1031, 1945.
20. Pont A, Williams PL, Azhan S: Ketoconazole blocks testosterone synthesis. *Arch Intern Med* 142:2137, 1982.
21. Drago SE, Rohner T, Santer R: Aminoglutethimide medical adrenalectomy for advanced prostate cancer. *J Urol* 115:170, 1976.
22. Plowman PN, Perry LA, Chard T: Androgen suppression by hydrocortisone without aminoglutethimide in orchiectomized men with prostate cancer. *Br J Urol* 59:255, 1987.

23. Isaacs JT, Coffrey D: Adaption versus selection as the mechanism responsible for the relapse of prostatic cancer to androgen ablation therapy as studied in the Dunning R-3327-H adenocarcinoma. *Cancer Res* 41:5070, 1981.
24. Labrie F, Dupont A, Belanger A, et al: New concepts of the androgen sensitivity of prostate cancer. *Prog Clin Biol Res* 243A:145, 1987.
25. Beland G, Mostafa E, Yves F, et al: Total androgen ablation: Canadian experience. *Urol Clin North Am* 18:75–82, 1991.
26. Denis L, Moura JL, Bono A: Gorerelin acetate and flutamide versus bilateral orchiectomy: a phase III EORTC trial (30853). *Urology* 42:119–130, 1993.
27. Crawford DE, Nabors WL: Total androgen ablation: American experience. *Urol Clin North Am* 18:55–63, 1991.
28. Crawford ED, DeAntonio EP, Labie F, et al: Endocrine therapy of prostate cancer: optimal form and appropriate timing. *J Clin Endocrinol Metab* 80(4):1062–1066, 1995.
29. Catalona WJ: Management of cancer of the prostate. *N Engl J Med* 331:996–1004, 1994.
30. Yagoda A, Petrylak D: Cytotoxic chemotherapy for advanced hormone resistant prostate cancer. *Cancer* (Suppl)71(3):1098–1109, 1993.
31. Detreus F, Logothetis CJ, Samuels ML, et al: Continuous infusion of vinblastine for advanced hormone refractory prostate cancer. *Cancer Treat Rep* 69:885–886, 1985.
32. Scher HI, Curley T, Gilles N, et al: Trimetrexate in prostatic cancer: preliminary observations of the use of the prostate specific antigen and acid phosphatase as a marker in measurable hormone refractory disease. *J Clin Oncol* 8:1830–1838, 1990.
33. Yagoda A, Smith JA, Soloway MS, et al: Phase II study of estramustine phosphate in advanced hormone-refractory prostate cancer with increasing prostate specific antigen levels. Am Urol Assoc Annual Meeting 1991, Abstract #686. *J Urol* 145:384A, 1991.
34. Eisenberg MA: Chemotherapy for prostate cancer. In Wittes RE (ed): Consensus Development Conference on the Management of Clinically Localized Prostate Cancer. NCI Monographs. No. 7. Washington, DC, Government Printing Office, 1988, pp 151–153.
35. Seidman AD, Scher HI, Petrylak D, et al: Estramustine and vinblastine: use of prostate specific antigen as a clinical trial end point for hormone refractory prostatic cancer. *J Urol* 147: 931–934, 1992.
36. Myers C, Cooper M, Stein C, et al: Suramin: a novel growth factor antagonist with activity in hormone refractory metastatic prostate cancer. *J Clin Oncol* 10:881–889, 1992.
37. Keen CW: Half-body radiotherapy in the management of metastatic carcinoma of the prostate. *J Urol* 123:713, 1980.
38. Blake GM, Zugavovic MA, McEwan AJ, et al: Strontium-89 therapy: strontium kinetics in disseminated carcinoma of the prostate. *Eur J Nucl Med* 12:447–454, 1986.
39. Crawford DE, Kozlowski JM, Debrync FM, et al: The use of strontium-89 for palliation of pain from bone metastases associated with hormone-refractory prostate cancer. *Urology* 44(4): 481–485, 1994.
40. Kelly WK, Scher HI: Prostate specific antigen decline after antiandrogen withdrawal: the flutamide withdrawal syndrome. *J Urol* 149:607–609, 1993.

11

Hormone Refractory Prostate Cancer

Paul F. Schellhammer
Gregg R. Eure

Although the majority of patients with metastatic prostate cancer will respond to androgen deprivation, almost all patients will eventually relapse. The mechanism of androgen resistance remains uncertain.[1] Potential mechanisms include clonal selection of androgen independent cells, oncogene activation of androgen independent pathways, loss of suppressor genes, and/or androgen receptor alterations.

Most patients will succumb to their disease within 1 to 2 years of development of hormone refractory disease. Currently there is no standard treatment approach.

There are major difficulties encountered in analyzing treatment outcomes for hormone refractory prostate cancer. The definitions of hormone refractory disease differ significantly and the criteria for response are variable. Definitions include patients who manifest (1) symptomatic disease progression, (2) progressive imaging abnormalities, or (3) rise in prostate specific antigen (PSA) in the absence of symptoms or radiologic progression. In hormone-naive metastatic prostate cancer, patient subgroups with variable extent of osseous involvement are associated with different outcomes. A similar staging system in hormone refractory disease has been proposed. This staging system separates osseous disease and visceral disease by extent and predicts differences in response to treatment regimens.[2] Therefore, trials that do not precisely define populations treated and studied are difficult to interpret.

Additionally, the definitions of response to treatment of hormone refractory disease, until recently, have been limited to documentation of improvement of subjective symptoms and to the difficult interpretation of bone scan changes. Currently PSA can serve as a surrogate marker for disease activity. Some difficulties with using PSA as a surrogate marker include the fact that an agent may selectively destroy PSA-producing cells while not affecting more undifferentiated cells which do not produce PSA or may decrease PSA production without cell kill. Furthermore, after androgen deprivation, the dynamics of PSA production are significantly altered. No specific criteria have been established to identify a meaningful PSA response with therapy for hormone refractory disease. Kelly et al.[3] and Seidman et al.[4] have reported that patients achieving a ≥50% reduction in PSA in clinical trials of chemotherapy in hormone refractory cancer experienced a significantly longer median survival.

In 1993, Scher and Kelly[5] reported a group of patients who had initiated complete androgen blockade and presented for further treatment secondary to disease progression. The antiandrogen flutamide was discontinued. It was noted that follow-up PSA levels had decreased and that some patients experienced subjective and objective improvement. Dupont et al.[6] confirmed this paradoxical response. Therefore, before initiating any protocol for hormone refractory disease treated with maximum androgen blockade, the antiandrogen needs to be discontinued to assess the possibility of a "flutamide withdrawal syndrome." This provides an opportunity for disease regression with the simplest of maneuvers and also validates the PSA profile that follows institution of further therapy.

EXTERNAL BEAM RADIATION (EBR)

EBR, the traditional modality for pain palliation for hormone refractory prostate cancer, is delivered to one or two select areas identified as painful, "spot radiation," or, if pain sites are numerous, by half-body or whole-body techniques. An alternate delivery by radiopharmaceuticals will be more frequently employed in the future.

The mechanism of pain relief after EBR or radiopharmaceuticals is not clearly established. Pain relief can be rapid and dramatic and this immediate outcome is difficult to explain on the basis of tumor cell mass shrinkage. Bone destruction associated with cancer has been linked with osteoblastic activity which can be induced by a number of cytokines such as tumor necrosis factor (TNF), interleukin-1 (IL-1), and IL-6. The lymphocyte, which is responsible for the production of cytokines, is a very radiation-sensitive cell. Its destruction at the tumor site and the ensuing reduction in cytokine production may be responsible for immediate pain relief.

A large prospective randomized study of radiation therapy for bone metastases was conducted by the Radiation Therapy Oncology Group (RTOG) in Study 7,402 which compared 4,050 rad over 3 weeks to 2,000 rad over 1 week for patients with solitary osseous metastases.[7] Pain relief was noted in the first 4 weeks of treatment and 54% eventually obtained complete pain relief. There were no significant differences between the treatment schedules and therefore short courses are convenient and cost-effective. RTOG trial 7,810 evaluated single-dose hemibody radiation for the palliation of multiple bone metastases.[8] Approximately 73% of patients achieved pain relief and 20% experienced complete pain relief. The safest and most effective dosages were 600 Cy for upper half-body radiation and 800 Cy for lower half-body and mid-body radiation. Our experience with 31 patients treated by half-body radiation at Eastern Virginia Medical School provided palliation of pain until death for 82% of patients receiving upper and 67% of patients receiving lower half radiation.

RTOG 8,206 evaluated whether the addition of single-dose half-body radiation (hemibody irradiation [HBI]) to standard local field radiation was more effective than local field radiation alone.[9] Among 499 patients studied, the time to disease progression was delayed significantly in the local plus HBI arm and the study concluded that HBI delayed the appearance of new metastases and the progression of existing metastases. The introduction of radiopharmaceuticals will offer a more convenient avenue of "systemic" radiation delivery.

RADIOPHARMACEUTICALS

Phosphorus-32 was first introduced for the treatment of metastatic prostate cancer and was the only available agent until the FDA approval of strontium-89 in 1993. An excellent review by Silberstein[10] outlines the results of ^{32}P therapy in 28 studies. While ^{32}P was effective in providing pain relief, the major side effect of bone marrow suppression, based on the high-energy beta emission of the isotope, limited its application. Other therapeutic isotopes, namely strontium-89 (^{89}Sr), samarium-153 (^{153}Sm), and rhenium-186 (^{186}Re) have lower energy emissions. Like ^{32}P, ^{89}Sr localizes to bone by an exchange with the calcium component of hydroxy appetite. Re and Sm, however, are conjugated to a ligand which localizes in bone. After ^{89}Sr, the cytopenia may persist for as long as 3 months. The half-lives of ^{186}Re and ^{153}Sm are much shorter and, therefore, only 1 to 2 weeks of bone marrow suppression are noted.

^{89}Sr has been extensively studied in prospective randomized trials. A multicenter trial[11] (trans-Canada study) randomized 126 patients with hormone refractory prostate cancer to EBR alone or EBR followed by adjuvant ^{89}Sr. EBR and ^{89}Sr produced a statistically significant reduction in pain score, reduction in analgesic therapy, and a reduction in the number of subsequent new sites of pain. The ^{89}Sr arm also performed more favorably in quality of life assessment and reduction in PSA and prostatic acid phosphatase levels. Survival was not affected.

A cost analysis was done as part of the trans-Canada study. It showed that treatment with ^{89}Sr produced meaningful reductions in lifetime management cost in patients with advanced prostate cancer by reducing need for further treatment and decreasing requirements for hospital admission.[12]

Novel approaches using ^{89}Sr therapy are being tested. A phase II study tested ^{89}Sr in combination with low-dose infusion cisplatinum, a radiosensitizing chemotherapeutic agent, and has reported improvements in pain relief and significant reductions in prostate specific antigen, alkaline phosphatase, and lactase dehydrogenase.[13] Radiopharmaceuticals may be used in combination with biphosphinates which enhance retention of radioisotopes at the site of bone metastases. Colony-stimulating factors may reduce the marrow suppression associated with radiopharmaceuticals.

CYTOTOXIC CHEMOTHERAPY

In the past 25 years there have been many trials using both single agents and multidrug regimens for patients with hormone refractory disease. Review of the available data by Eisenberger has shown limited partial and complete responses without any significant increase in survival.[14] Yagoda and Petrylak confirmed this finding by tabulating a complete and partial remission rate of 6.5%[15] among 3,148 patients compiled from a number of series. Only six agents had an objective response rate >10%. The most promising of these were estramustine alone and in combination with vinblastine, vinblastine by bolus and continuous infusion, and trimetrexate. Sella et al. recently reported PSA response to a phase II trial which combines ketoconazole with weekly doxorubicin.[16]

Estramustine phosphate (PO_4) links estradiol and nitrogen mustard. Estramustine phosphate has been compared to standard hormonal manipulations and found to be comparable in efficacy. Recently estramustine has been combined with vinblastine or etoposide. Vinblastine inhibits microtubule formation and estramustine binds to microtubule-associated proteins. In vitro studies show additive antimitotic activity. Trials using estramustine and vinblastine have reported 50–60% declines in PSA levels, pain relief in 43–66%, and partial tumor responses. Using estramustine and etoposide in a preliminary trial of 20 patients, Pienta reported five patients with stable disease and 11 with partial remissions.[17] These results support the investigation of other microtubular inhibitors, such as Taxol.

SECOND LINE HORMONAL AGENTS

Ketoconazole, an imidazole derivative and therapeutic antifungal agent, blocks the cytochrome P-450 biosynthesis of testosterone. At a dose of 400 mg 3 times a day, castrate levels can be reached within 24 hours and it is therefore effective in urgent initial first line therapy for metastatic disease.[18] As therapy in hormone refractory disease it blocks adrenal androgens and may benefit those patients who have not undergone total androgen blockade as first line therapy. It also has been postulated to have a direct in vivo cytotoxic effect on prostate cancer cells.[19] Clinical studies, however, have not been encouraging. Jubelirer and Hogan noted complete and partial responses in less than 1% and 14% of patients respectively.[20] Chodak reported a response in 3 of 15 patients treated with both ketoconazole and prednisone.[21] Side effects which include gastrointestinal intolerance, weakness, and adrenal insufficiency limit therapy. Survival has not been prolonged.

Stilbestrol diphosphate is a biologically inactive water-soluble estrogen that has been available since 1946. It can be injected intravenously in large doses where it has shown direct cytotoxic activity against prostate carcinoma.[22] The compound is dephosphorylated by acid phosphatase and thereby is converted to the active estrogen, diethylstilbestrol (DES). It is believed that the higher serum doses by intravenous injection account for the direct cytotoxicity that was not demonstrable in previous studies using the oral route.

Droz et al. recently completed a phase I trial that used a 4 gm per day infusion over $3\frac{1}{2}$ hr for a duration up to 10 days.[23] Nausea and emesis were the dose-limiting side effect. Ferro et al. noted improvement in pain, mobility, and analgesic requirements in 22 of 29 patients with hormone refractory disease.[24] Thirteen showed significant falls in PSA levels albeit short-lived. They recommended 1,140 mg (four vials of 285 mg) once or twice daily for 7–10 days.

Progestational agents such as megestrol acetate, hydroxyprogesterone caproate, and medrogestone function by inhibiting pituitary luteinizing hormone (LH) secretion and decreasing both plasma testosterone and 4-dihydrotestosterone (DHT). Most also have androgen receptor antagonist activity. They have produced only minimal partial responses and concern exists regarding potential stimulatory effect by their androgenic properties.[25]

Aminoglutethimide suppresses adrenal androgen production by blocking cytochrome P450 conversion of cholesterol. At high doses it can completely suppress adrenal function and therefore requires hydrocortisone replacement. In fact, some of its clinical benefits may be related to the hydrocortisone effect rather than the blockade of adrenal androgen production. Plowman et al. reported that similar response rates can be obtained with hydrocortisone alone.[26]

A study by Sartor et al. reported an 80% decline in PSA for more than 4 weeks in 14 of 29 patients with hormone refractory disease treated with aminoglutethimide therapy in combination with flutamide withdrawal.[27] Whether withdrawal or addition of aminoglutethimide was operative is conjectural.

Although there have been some objective and subjective responses reported with aminoglutethimide therapy, there has been no significant effect of survival. Side effects include hypothyroidism, lethargy, rash, and less commonly, severe pancytopenia.

NOVEL THERAPIES: SIGNAL TRANSDUCTION GROWTH FACTORS AND DIFFERENTIATING AGENTS

A complex array of biochemical pathways generate intracellular signals that control gene expression and cell function. These processes, known as *signal transduction*, are typically initiated by the activation of membrane receptors. Due to alterations in the receptors and attendant altered or exaggerated responses, neoplasia can result. Because aberrant signal transduction is one of the hallmarks of malignantly transformed cells, changes in tumor cell signaling pathways with novel drugs may offer new approaches to the treatment of cancer. Since signal transduction therapy can be totally unassociated with hormonal regulation and the effects of androgen deprivation, signal transduction therapy might be a potential avenue of treatment for hormone refractory disease. Intracellular calcium regulates signaling events and is required for cell proliferation. Carboxymidotriazole (CAI) is a synthetic drug that disrupts calcium homeostasis. In vitro, using concentrations achievable and tolerable in vivo, there was inhibition of cellular proliferation in the DU145, LNCAP, and PC3 lines (Wasilenko, Schellhammer, unpublished data). Other drugs aimed at signal transduction alterations are under investigation. A trial reported by Myers et al. used suramin in patients with hormone refractory disease and found pain relief in 71% and 50% reduction in PSA levels in 55% of the patients.[28] Patients with greater than 75% decline in serum PSA by week 8 of therapy had an 85% probability of survival at 1 year. Toxicity has been a critical issue. In Myers' study, there was a 5% mortality related secondarily to drug toxicity.

The growth factor inhibitor, somatostatin, and its more potent analogs have shown promising activity presumptively by blocking autocrine tumor cell activity. Schally et al. reported a direct antiproliferative effect of somatostatin analogs in experimental cell line in animal models.[29] When used as first line therapy in conjunction with luteinizing hormone–releasing hormone (LH-RH) agonists there is a delay in development of hormone refractory disease. Clinical trials have shown only limited or partial responses.[30] Toxicity is minimal.

A potentially useful molecule for the treatment of hormone refractory prostate cancer is phenylacetate (NaPA).[31] It acts as a differentiating agent, inducing tumors to reverse their malignant direction. Phenylacetate has been tested in vitro against the human prostate cancer cell lines PC3, DU145, and LNCAP and has demonstrated the ability to suppress proliferation and revert the cell lines to a nonmalignant phenotype. It also has shown the ability to act in an additive manner when combined with suramin. The combination promises tumor responses possible with significantly lower doses of suramin.

Liarozole is a benzimidazole compound which is related to ketoconazole but unlike ketoconazole, it does not modify adrenal androgen or cortisol levels. Its efficacy and toxicity are related to its ability to raise endogenous levels of retinoic acid probably by binding to the cytochrome P450 moiety responsible for retinoic acid catabolism.[32] In preclinical testing, the compound was found to be effective in reducing the growth of hormone refractory clones of the DU145 prostate carcinoma. In a phase I/II trial of 44 patients with metastatic hormone refractory prostate cancer, objective responses occurred in approximately 30% of patients with measurable disease, and a prostate specific antigen reduction of 50% or more was noted in half of the patients. Subjective pain relief was common. The primary toxicities are mucositis, dermatitis, and nausea.

CONCLUSION

Despite an increase in public awareness, medical interests, and screening efforts, a significant proportion of men continue to present with metastatic and advanced disease. Management of these patients following escape from hormonal therapy remains unsatisfactory. Current research is focused on new cellular and molecular aspects of prostate cancer with new opportunities for intervention. As the search continues, it remains important to continue to offer patients available palliative therapies with attention to quality of life.

The Office of Alternative Medicine (OAM) has joined with the National Cancer Institute (NCI) to sponsor scientific trials to generate data to either support or refute claims of new products for the treatment of cancer, such as shark cartilage. The aim is to share expertise in random clinical trials with alternative medicine practitioners. Results from these trials will generate significant public interest for advocates of alternative therapy.

REFERENCES

1. McConnell JD: Physiologic basis of endocrine therapy for prostatic cancer. *Urol Clin North Am* 18(1):1–13, 1991.
2. Logothetis CJ, Samuels ML, von Eschenbach AC, et al: Doxorubicin, mitomycin-C, and 5-fluorouracil (DMF) in the treatment of metastatic hormonal refractory adenocarcinoma of the prostate, with a note on the staging of metastatic prostate cancer. *J Clin Oncol* 1:368–379, 1983.
3. Kelly WK, Scher HI, Mazumdar M, et al: Prostate-specific antigen as a measure of disease outcome in metastatic hormone-refractory prostate cancer. *J Clin Oncol* 11:607, 1993.
4. Seidman AD, Scher HI, Petrylak D, et al: Estramustine and vinblastine: use of prostate specific antigen as a clinical trial end point for hormone refractory prostate cancer. *J Urol* 147:931, 1992.
5. Scher HI, Kelly WK: Flutamide withdrawal syndrome: its impact on clinical trials in hormone-refractory prostate cancer. *J Clin Oncol* 11:1566–1572, 1993.
6. Dupont A, Gomez J-L, Cusan L, et al: Response to flutamide withdrawal in advanced prostate cancer in progression under combination therapy. *J Urol* 150:908–913, 1993.
7. Tong D, Gillick L, Hendrickson FR: The palliation of symptomatic osseous metastases: final results of the study by the Radiation Therapy Oncology Group. *Cancer* 55:1468–1472, 1985.

8. Salazar OM, Rubin P, Hendrickson F, et al: Single dose half-body irradiation for palliation of multiple bone metastases from solid tumors. *Cancer* 58:29–36, 1986.

9. Poulter CA, Cosmatos D, Rubin P, et al: A report of RTOG 8206: a phase III study of whether the addition of single dose hemibody irradiation to standard fractionated local field irradiation is more effective than local field irradiation alone in the treatment of symptomatic osseous metastases. *Int J Radiat Oncol Biol Phys* 23:207–214, 1992.

10. Silberstein EB: The treatment of painful osseous metastases with phosphorus-32–labeled phosphates. *Semin Oncol* 20(3):10–21, 1993.

11. Porter AT, McEwan AJB, Powe JE, et al: Results of a randomized phase-III trial to evaluate the efficacy of strontium-89 adjuvant to local field external beam irradiation in the management of endocrine resistant metastatic prostate cancer. *Int J Radiat Oncol Biol Phys* 25:805–813, 1993.

12. McEwan AJB, Amyotte GA, McGowan DG, et al: A retrospective analysis of the cost effectiveness of treatment with Metastron® (^{89}Sr-chloride) in patients with prostate cancer metastatic to bone. *Nuclear Med Commun* 15:499–504, 1994.

13. Mertens WC, Porter AT, Reid RH, et al: Strontium-89 and low-dose infusion of cisplatin for patients with hormone refractory prostate carcinoma metastatic to bone: a preliminary report. *J Nuclear Med* 33:1437–1443, 1992.

14. Eisenberger MA: Chemotherapy for prostate cancer. *NCI Monogr* 7:151–163, 1988.

15. Yagoda A, Petrylak D: Cytotoxic chemotherapy for advanced hormone-resistant prostate cancer. *Cancer* 71:1098–1109, 1993.

16. Sella A, Kilbourn R, Amato R, et al: Phase II study of ketoconazole combined with weekly doxorubicin in patients with androgen-independent prostate cancer. *J Clin Oncol* 12(4): 683–688, 1994.

17. Pienta KJ, Lehr JE: Inhibition of prostate cancer growth by estramustine and etoposide: evidence for interaction at the nuclear matrix. *J Urol* 149:1622–1625, 1993.

18. Lowe FC, Bamberger MH: Indications for use of ketoconazole in management of metastatic prostate cancer. *Urology* 36(6):541–545, 1990.

19. Eichenberger T, Trachtenberg P: Ketoconazole: a possible direct cytotoxic effect on prostate carcinoma cells. *J Urol* 141:190–191, 1989.

20. Jubelirer SJ, Hogan T: High dose ketoconazole for the treatment of hormone refractory metastatic prostate carcinoma: 16 cases and review of the literature. *J Urol* 142:89–91, 1989.

21. Gerber GS, Chodak GW: Prostate specific antigen for assessing response to ketoconazole and prednisone in patients with hormone refractory metastatic prostate cancer. *J Urol* 144: 1177–1179, 1990.

22. Ferro MA: Use of intravenous stilbestrol diphosphate in patients with prostatic carcinoma refractory to conventional hormonal manipulation. *Urol Clin North Am* 18(1):139, 1991.

23. Droz JP, De Smedt J, Kattan F, et al: Phase I trial of high-dose fosfestrol in hormone-refractory adenocarcinoma of the prostate. *Prostate* 24:62–66, 1994.

24. Ferro CA, Gillatt D, Symes MO, et al: High dose intravenous estrogen therapy in advanced prostatic carcinoma: use of prostate specific antigen as a serum marker. *Urology* 24:134–138, 1989.

25. Mahler C, Denis L: Management of relapsing disease in prostate cancer. *Cancer* 70:329–334, 1992.

26. Plowman PN, Perry LA, Chard T: Androgen suppression by hydrocortisone without aminoglutethimide in orchiectomised men with prostate cancer. *Br J Urol* 59:255–257, 1987.

27. Sartor O, Cooper M, Weinberger M, et al: Surprising activity of flutamide withdrawal when

combined with aminoglutethimide, in treatment of "hormone refractory" prostate cancer. *J Natl Cancer Inst* 86(3):222–227, 1994.

28. Myers C, Cooper M, Stein C, et al: Suramin: a novel growth factor antagonist with activity in hormone-refractory metastatic prostate cancer. *J Clin Oncol* 10:881–889, 1992.
29. Pinski J, Halmos G, Schally AV: Somatostatin analog RC-160 and bombesin/gastrin-releasing peptide antagonist RC-3095 inhibit the growth of androgen-independent DU-145 human prostate cancer line in nude mice. *Cancer Lett* 7:189–196, 1993.
30. Dupont A, Boucher H, Cusan L: Octreotide and bromocriptine in patients with stage D2 prostate cancer who relapsed during treatment with flutamide and castration. *Eur J Cancer* 26:770–771, 1990.
31. Samid D, Shack S, Myers C: Selective growth arrest and phenotypic reversion of prostate cancer cells in vitro by nontoxic pharmacological concentrations of phenylacetate. *J Clin Invest* 91:2288–2295, 1993.
32. Stearns ME, Wang M, Fudge K: Liarozole and 13-*cis*-retinoic acid anti-prostatic tumor activity. *Cancer Res* 53:3073–3077, 1993.

12

Treatment of Postprostatectomy Incontinence and Impotence

Richard F. Labasky, M.D.

The good news of a probable cure of prostate cancer by a radical prostatectomy is frequently clouded by the reality of two common consequences of the surgery: incontinence and impotence (erectile dysfunction).[1–3] However, these problems can be successfully treated in almost all patients after a careful evaluation, and selection of therapy which balances the level of success that the patient desires with the risks he is willing to accept.

MECHANISMS OF CONTINENCE AND INCONTINENCE

Maintaining continence requires normal function by the three elements of the lower urinary tract—the bladder, the urethra, and the sensation. The normal bladder can maintain continence bladder by filling to normal volumes with little to no pressure rise; it can do this because of the viscoelastic properties of the bladder wall and suppression of detrusor contraction by inhibitory neurologic input. Thus, the bladder can cause incontinence if the pressures or volumes of the bladder are abnormal.

The urethra maintains continence by keeping the sphincter closed (competent) except during voiding. Incontinence occurs if one or more of the components of the sphincter (see Table 12.1) lose normal functional capability. The muscle layers are the most important elements. A smooth muscle layer with abundant α-adrenergic agonist receptors extends from the bladder neck to near the membranous urethra. The rhabdosphincter, a striated muscle composed mostly of fatigue-resistant, slow-twitch fibers, is located from the distal prostate gland through the membranous urethra. These muscles possess a resting

TABLE 12.1. Primary Elements of the Urethral Sphincter Mechanism Necessary to Maintain Continence

1.	A supple epithelium that coapts to form a urethral seal
2.	A surrounding vascular submucosal layer which provides further bulk and suppleness to the epithelial layer
3.	Muscle layers which contract to compress the inner submucosal and urethral epithelial layers
4.	Collagen and elastin within the submucosal and muscle layers
5.	Intact innervation of the muscle layers

tone essential to passive continence. Active continence is dependent upon the somatically innervated striated muscle of the external sphincter attached to the pelvic floor at the membranous urethra.[4]

Normal sensation function permits detection of bladder volume and pressure levels and initiation of proper sphincteric contraction to guard against incontinence.

Surgical alteration of the bladder, sphincter, or sensation can lead to incontinence. Thus, careful attention to surgical technique during radical prostatectomy to prevent incontinence has gained widespread attention. The most recent refinements in technique include careful maintenance of the structures of the anterior urethra and dorsal vein complex, precise apical dissection of the prostate to maintain maximum sphincter length, incorporation of the periurethral striated muscle to create an anatomic anastomosis, eversion of the bladder wall epithelium ensuring a watertight urethral anastomosis, careful tissue handling, and minimal dissection and coagulation around the bladder and urethra. Tubularization of the bladder neck may yield earlier restoration of continence without clear change in overall continence rates. The value of the cavernous nerve-sparing procedure in assisting continence is unclear.[2,4]

Some patients may be at greater risk for postprostatectomy incontinence because of preoperative conditions such as those who have had transurethral resection of the prostate or pelvic radiation, or those patients with diabetes, Parkinson's, lumbar disc or other neuromuscular disease, local tumor extension into the sphincter, and pre- or postoperative bladder neck contracture.[2,4]

While most patients are incontinent immediately after prostatectomy, most ultimately regain continence. At one year postoperatively the reported incontinence rates are 0 to 35% continuous or severe incontinence, and 2–23% milder incontinence. The extreme variability in the reported incidence of incontinence results from the inconsistent definitions of incontinence and the usually subjective nature of the assessments.[1,2,4,5]

The true etiology of postprostatectomy incontinence is rarely confirmed, leading to the incorrect assumption that incontinence is always a result of iatrogenic sphincter damage. In reality, detailed urodynamic analyses have shown that as many as 25–55% of patients with post radical prostatectomy incontinence have some element of detrusor dysfunction (low compliance or detrusor instability) which could contribute to the leakage.[5] Not recognizing the true cause of incontinence can have dramatic implications for therapy selection.

Evaluation and Classification of Incontinence

Treatment of incontinence after prostatectomy is based upon a basic evaluation which allows exclusion of morbid causes of the incontinence, such as recurrent or metastatic disease, and a clinical classification of the type of incontinence.[6] Reversible therapies directed toward achieving the patient's goals in managing the problem can then be initiated. More intensive tests such as cystoscopy and urodynamics can be performed to help confirm the etiology of the problem and permit precise direction of the therapy options.

A clinical classification of any patient's incontinence can be made based upon the patient's description of the incontinence, supplemented by other aspects of the medical history, an examination, and a simple set of tests. With this core evaluation, the patient's incontinence can be classified into one of five types of clinical incontinence: transient, overflow, continuous, stress, and urge. These types of incontinence and their causes are familiar to most urologists.[6]

Transient incontinence has an acute and recent onset, with a readily reversible cause; it is most commonly due to infection or a medication change. Overflow incontinence results from an inability to empty the bladder adequately because of urethral obstruction or loss of detrusor contractility. Continuous incontinence is urinary leakage which is unrelenting. After prostatectomy, it usually is due to loss of urethral sphincter competence (intrinsic sphincteric deficiency [ISD]). Stress incontinence results from less severe ISD. Urge incontinence occurs with a nonsuppressible need to urinate, most often due to uninhibited detrusor contractions (detrusor instability [DI] or hyperreflexia [DH]). Frequency and nocturia are common with urge incontinence.

EVALUATION OF INCONTINENCE

History

Generally, the patient will describe his incontinence in one of the ways noted above. The balance of the medical history should include information about the course, duration, and severity of the incontinence; preprostatectomy continence status; prior and present methods of therapy or hygiene and their results; irritative and obstructive voiding symptoms; other medical, surgical, and neurologic diagnoses; of symptoms focusing on the neurologic, musculoskeletal, and gastrointestinal systems.

Physical Examination

The physical examination helps exclude ISD, overflow, and neurologically induced incontinence. A tender suprapubic mass may be a distended bladder causing overflow incontinence. Observing incontinence with the patient at rest helps diagnose overflow or continuous incontinence. Incontinence with straining maneuvers helps diagnose stress incontinence. An abnormal rectal or lower extremity neurologic examination may indicate a neurologic abnormality causing incontinence.

TABLE 12.2. Indications for Cystoscopy in Evaluating Postprostatectomy Incontinence

1. To confirm suspected obstruction from stricture or bladder neck contracture
2. To confirm the diagnosis of ISD by seeing the urethra open from the bladder neck to the bulbous urethra
3. To assess the length and suppleness of the remaining sphincter for injection of periurethral bulking agents
4. To rule out foreign bodies, stones, or tumor spread into the trigone in patients with severe irritative symptoms and urgency incontinence

Complementary Tests

A urinalysis and serum creatinine rule out infections, hematuria, glucosuria, or occult renal disease that may cause transient, overflow, or urgency incontinence. A residual urine check is essential to rule out overflow incontinence. Passing an 18-French catheter rules out anatomic obstruction causing urgency or overflow incontinence. Cystoscopy can be useful for several reasons (see Table 12.2).

"Eyeball urodynamics" can help confirm ISD or urgency incontinence. After passing a catheter and measuring residual urine, the bladder is slowly filled by gravity via the catheter attached to a catheter tip syringe. As the bladder fills, patient urgency with a rise in the water column may be consistent with urgency incontinence. When the patient feels full, the capacity is noted and the catheter is removed. Leakage without pressure rise or straining indicates continuous incontinence from severe ISD; leakage requiring straining, in any position, indicates stress incontinence and less severe ISD. If the water column is high (>20 cm) at capacity and leak occurs after catheter removal, overflow incontinence from low bladder compliance may be present.[6]

Radiographic tests such as a cystogram or voiding cystourethrogram could be useful in preoperative planning but are not essential.

URODYNAMIC CLASSIFICATION

A formal urodynamic evaluation is "eyeball urodynamics" performed with precise data measurement and recording equipment. The measurements allow a urodynamic classification of the patient's incontinence which is usually more precise than that obtained from the basic evaluation. The general indications for urodynamic evaluations for incontinence are summarized in Table 12.3.[6–8]

The most important caveat about the appropriate and valid use of urodynamics is that the tests should duplicate as closely as possible the incontinence that the patient is experiencing to confirm the true etiology. If the test does not duplicate such symptoms, the test has not been adequately performed; if the test induces abnormalities which the patient does not usually experience, the findings are generally considered artifact and not clinically significant. A discussion of the technical details and considerations in performing and interpreting urodynamics is beyond the scope of this chapter but can be found elsewhere.[6,8]

TABLE 12.3. Indications for Urodynamics Evaluations in Patients with Postprostatectomy Incontinence

1. Failed medical therapies
2. Failed surgical therapies
3. Consideration for surgical therapy, especially as the first therapy step
4. Incontinence associated with known or potential neurologic causes
5. Complex or combined clinical types or causes of incontinence
6. Contradictory, confusing, or noncontributory history, physical examination, or basic tests, leading to an inability to make a good clinical classification of the incontinence

Cystometrogram

The cystometrogram (CMG) is the most useful urodynamic test in evaluation of incontinence since it can detect the primary causes of postprostatectomy incontinence: abnormal detrusor pressures (DI or DH, or low compliance); ISD; and altered sensation.

Incontinence from DI usually presents as urge incontinence. Low compliance may present as overflow, urge, or stress incontinence. After prostatectomy, the most common causes of DI are: idiopathic; infections; urethral obstruction; bladder stones, foreign bodies or tumors; DH results from spinal cord metastases, or concomitant neurologic diseases. Low compliance is caused by pelvic nerve or spinal cord metastases or injury, urethral obstruction, and possibly by damage of detrusor neural input during radical prostatectomy.

Incontinence due to ISD may present as continuous or stress incontinence. ISD often has an iatrogenic cause. However, some preoperative incompetence may be unmasked when a larger portion of the sphincter is removed during a routine prostatectomy. Formal urodynamics permits measurement of the amount of intra-abdominal pressure needed to induce stress incontinence, a pressure now termed the Valsalva leak point pressure (VLPP). The VLPP is increased by artifact such as larger catheter sizes during the test and greater urethral narrowing due to such problems as bladder neck contractures. VLPP also lacks correlation with incontinence severity. Thus, the value of VLPP in postprostatectomy incontinence is unclear.

Bladder sensation can be reduced by diabetes, neurologic disease, or chronic retention; it can lead to retention or reduced ability of the patient to feel detrusor pressure rises and to guard against incontinence. Reduced sensation can lead to overflow, continuous, or urge incontinence. Increased sensation can cause irritative symptoms and urge incontinence; it usually results from infection, tumor spread to the trigone, or obstruction.

Complementary Urodynamics Tests

Voiding cystometry (pressure/flow study) helps confirm whether overflow incontinence is caused by obstruction or by detrusor acontractility/areflexia. Obstruction may also cause urge incontinence. Uroflowmetry, electromyography (EMG), and urethral pressure profilometry have no unique clinical utility in diagnosing postprostatectomy incontinence. Performing the CMG or pressure/flow study with simultaneous fluoroscopy (videourodynamics) can correlate the physiologic measurements of urodynamics with the anatomy of the lower urinary tract but is not routinely needed in the evaluation of postprostatectomy incontinence.[6,8]

TREATMENT OF INCONTINENCE

There are five main principles for management of incontinence after radical prostatectomy: (1) the therapy selected should be based upon the conclusions reached in the evaluation of the patient, not upon assumptions or guesses about the probable cause of post-prostatectomy incontinence; (2) therapy should be selected based upon the treatment goals of the patient in terms of the desired rapidity and thoroughness of the treatment result; (3) it usually is most reasonable to use simple, reversible techniques first and then escalate to more invasive techniques if these fail; (4) the simple, reversible therapies can be started at any time after prostatectomy; (5) no surgical therapy should be attempted for approximately one year after prostatectomy to allow for potential spontaneous resolution of incontinence to occur.

Therapy options that should be presented to all patients with postprostatectomy incontinence with any etiology can be divided into three main categories: behavioral, medical, and surgical.[7,9] With any therapy, encouragement and positive reinforcement can improve a patient's compliance and outlook, especially in the early postoperative period since spontaneous resolution of incontinence ultimately will occur is most patients.

Behavioral Therapies

Behavioral therapies help modify the patient's behavior and activities to improve or manage the incontinence.

Altering Fluid Intake and Voiding Patterns

The appropriateness of reducing fluid intake or increasing the frequency of voiding to reduce the volume of incontinence can be assessed with a fluid intake/output record. Patients may also notice that certain drinks or food worsen the incontinence; these should be avoided. Timed-voiding patterns also can be useful.

Collection Devices

A variety of devices are available to allow collection of the urinary leakage. Simple techniques such as rolled up tissues, clothes, towels, and other homemade devices may work just as well as commercially available pads or diapers. There are urinary collectors that attach with adhesive to the underwear and fit over the penis and absorb leakage. A condom catheter can be used to collect large volumes of leakage without the need to change the device throughout the day. External clamps can provide gentle pressure to the urethra to produce intermittent continence; they should be released every 3 hr. The patient using these approaches must be advised about techniques to limit or treat penile skin and urethral damage.

Exercises

Pelvic floor exercises (Kegel exercises) can increase the closure capability of the voluntary sphincter. Success with the exercises often is better if the patient is given instructions on how to perform them prior to surgery so that he can begin the exercises as soon as the catheter has been removed. Patients often need coaching and supplementary instruction on how to perform the exercises; printed materials and audiocassettes which can assist in this way are available from Help for Incontinent People (HIP, phone: 800-BLADDER [252-3337]). Patients can experience a 30–40% improvement with these techniques for stress incontinence and ISD.

Electrical Stimulation

Providing stimulation to the pelvic floor and sphincteric muscles using skin or anal plug electrical simulators, has the potential of improving urinary continence. After starting in the office or clinic setting, patients can then use devices of this type at home to continue the muscle strengthening process. Successes of up to 45% have been achieved in some studies for stress and urge incontinence, DI/DH, and ISD.

Biofeedback

The ability of the patient to actually see or hear, and thus improve, the quality of the contractions he is achieving with pelvic floor muscle exercises is the principle behind the potential success of biofeedback therapy. Contraction quality is assessed with EMG probes placed on the perianal skin or within the rectum. These techniques can be used in conjunction with electrical stimulation and Kegel exercises to enhance their success.

Catheterization

Patients with overflow incontinence with retention because of detrusor acontractility or areflexia can use intermittent self-catheterization to empty the bladder. Indwelling urethral or suprapubic catheterization can also be used for any cause of incontinence, though they usually are not appropriate considering the variety of other successful options.

Medical Therapy

Medications can be extremely useful in treating postprostatectomy incontinence. Selection of the medications depends upon whether the incontinence is a consequence of bladder or sphincteric dysfunction.

Medications can improve detrusor storage characteristics by improving instability/hyperreflexia or low compliance. The anticholinergic agent propantheline can be taken on an empty stomach in doses from 7.5 mg (one-half of a regular tablet) to 30 mg, once a day to four times a day. Smooth muscle relaxants such as oxybutinin (2.5–5 mg, once a day to four times a day) or dicyclomine (10–20 mg, once a day to three times a day) can also be beneficial. Side effects typical of these medications include dry mouth and constipation; these can be managed by chewing gum or sucking on candies, and with generous use of fiber, stool softeners, and laxatives. These medications are contraindicated with narrow-angle glaucoma.

To improve sphincter closure tone (ISD), inexpensive, over-the-counter α-adrenergic agonist medications such as phenylpropanolamine (25–75 mg, once a day to twice daily) and pseudoephedrine (30–60 mg twice a day to four times a day) can be used to increase contraction of the sphincter smooth muscle. A trial at the highest tolerable doses for 2 to 4 weeks is reasonable. Patients with hypertension, hyperthyroidism, or cardiac disease should have clearance from their primary care physician before using these medications.

Imipramine can also be used for treating detrusor or sphincter dysfunction using 10–25 mg once a day to four times a day.

In using these medications to correct bladder or sphincter dysfunction, it usually is necessary to start with low doses but to be willing to push the dosage high enough to cause notable side effects before they are likely to be effective against incontinence. Care must be taken to titrate the doses according to the patient's other medical problems and medications.

Surgical Therapy

When behavioral or medical therapies fail, or the patient wishes to have the greatest likelihood of regaining substantial continence, surgical therapy is an excellent option.

Treating Bladder Dysfunction

In a few rare instances, incontinence because of detrusor dysfunction will not respond adequately to medications. In these situations an augmentation enterocystoplasty may be considered, and will be very successful. The suitability of a partial detrusormyomectomy (autoaugmentation) is still being studied. The procedure certainly is much more difficult to perform after a prostatectomy.

Treating Sphincter Dysfunction

To correct incontinence due to poor sphincteric coaptation (ISD) two therapies are available: periurethral bulking agents and the artificial urinary sphincter. The primary caveat that applies to treatment of sphincter dysfunction surgically is that any detrusor dysfunction should be diagnosed and treated first. Failure to follow this sequence can lead to persistent incontinence, possibly unnecessary sphincteric surgery and upper urinary tract compromise, and an unhappy patient and frustrated urologist.

The only agent approved for use to provide sphincteric bulk is glutaraldehyde-crosslinked bovine collagen (Contigen, from Bard Urological). The substance is indicated for use for incontinence from ISD of at least one year duration. It is injected with cystoscopic guidance under the urethral epithelium from the bladder neck to the membranous urethra. Urethral lidocaine anesthetic usually is adequate. Most men require approximately three injections to achieve initial improvement in the incontinence, or dryness; the injections must be repeated in most patients in later months or years to restore the initial benefit obtained. Overall, about one-third of patients initially can become dry, and about another one-half will have some improved continence. The primary complications are limited to allergic reactions, infections, and retention in a small percentage of patients.

Collagen injections seem to be most effective in men with milder stress rather than continuous incontinence. Patients with longer and more supple sphincteric urethras also seem to respond better than patients with shorter lengths or urethral scarring.

Periurethral injection of autologous fat has been attempted. Success with postprostatectomy incontinence has been minimal. Collagen implantation has supplanted the use of polytetrafluoroethylene (Teflon) injection because of the risk of Teflon particle migration, absence of FDA approval of Teflon for this application, and greater difficulty in injecting the Teflon.

The artificial urinary sphincter has been a mainstay of correction of ISD for more than a decade. Implantation requires a general or spinal anesthetic but success rates (dryness, or leakage requiring no more than two pads/day) of at least 90% have been achieved. Successes are less in patients with histories of bladder neck contracture, radiation therapy, or metastatic cancer. Revisions of the device are needed in about one-third of all patients because of mechanical failure, cuff erosion, urethral atrophy, and infection. Smaller cuff sizes (4.0 cm) are now available to improve coaptation with smaller urethral calibers. Lower pressure reservoirs (51–60 cm water) and deactivation of the system at night can reduce the risk of atrophy or erosion in patients with prior radiation therapy or prior atrophy.

Incision of a bladder neck contracture can be performed at the same time as a collagen injection if the extent of the contracture incision will not compromise the ability of the tissue to take up and hold the collagen. The appropriateness of incising a bladder neck contracture at the same time as placement of the artificial sphincter is uncertain though at least one recent study suggests that the risks of simultaneous procedures are not significantly increased.

EVALUATION AND TREATMENT OF IMPOTENCE (ERECTILE DYSFUNCTION)

Mechanisms of Erectile Function and Dysfunction

Normal erectile function is a complex phenomenon that requires intact endocrine, neurologic, vascular, and psychological function.[3] Abnormalities in any of these systems can cause erectile dysfunction. Only the endocrine system is not at risk from radical prostatectomy, but its function may be abnormal for other reasons before or after surgery.

Bilateral, and even unilateral injury to the cavernous nerves by radical prostatectomy can cause impotence. Even the best surgeons preserve potency after nerve-sparing prostatectomy in only 70% of patients overall, and in less than 25% in patients older than 70 years of age. Patients who fare best are: less than 50 years old (90% potency); older than 50 years of age with bilateral rather than unilateral nerve sparing; and those with no capsular penetration or seminal vesicle invasion by tumor. By one year after surgery, over 90% of those who will regain potency will have done so.[1,2] Other surgeons' potency preservation rates may be less because of differences in technique and in methods of assessing and reporting potency. Furthermore, some men with borderline normal erectile function before prostatectomy, or with vascular, neurologic disease or diabetes might be rendered totally impotent by the slightest trauma or cautery near the cavernous nerves. These same patients might be at risk from injury to accessory or main branches of the cavernous arteries. The depression and anxiety surrounding a cancer diagnosis, surgery, incomplete resection, or incontinence may be significant factors in altering normal sexual function.[3]

Evaluation of Erectile Dysfunction

Basic Evaluation

Evaluation of the patient with postprostatectomy erectile dysfunction should provide information about factors causing erectile dysfunction preoperatively or worsened postoperative function. The existing and prior libido, erectile rigidity, tumescence, and duration characterize the deficit. Delineating the relationship with the present sexual partner(s) is vital. A review of other illnesses and surgeries, and of the neurologic, vascular, genitourinary, gastrointestinal, and endocrine systems is important. Tobacco, alcohol, and medication use must be noted.

The physical exam should focus upon the peripheral pulses; testicular size and consistency; rectal exam; penile sensation; lower extremity reflexes; and anal sphincter tone, contractility, and bulbocavernosus reflex.

Blood tests should include serum chemistry and testosterone measurement if the patient had reduced erectile function before surgery, or if more than one year has elapsed since the prostatectomy.

Detailed Physiologic Testing

If there is a desire to obtain more detailed information about the probable etiology of the erectile dysfunction, detailed physiologic testing can be performed. These tests include nocturnal penile tumescence (NPT) monitoring, pharmacologic testing, ultrasound-pulsed Doppler study (duplex scan), cavernosometry/cavernosography, and arteriography. However, these are rarely performed after radical prostatectomy, and they are not necessary before initiating any of the nonsurgical therapy techniques. Even before placement of a penile prosthesis only NPT monitoring might be indicated to rule out psychogenic impotence.

Treatment of Erectile Dysfunction

Selection of the therapy for erectile dysfunction should be directed by the patient and his partner from the outset so that they can choose a successful technique they will use consistently. Issues for the couple to consider include likely success rate, risks, cost, and overall appeal or acceptability. In practice, most patients select one of the nonsurgical treatments first because of the concern about having another surgery and the potential risks and the costs of penile prostheses.[3]

Therapy for erectile dysfunction can begin whenever the patient is ready to do so after recovery from prostatectomy, perhaps as early as 3 months after surgery. For some men, it will be necessary to raise the question of erectile function on a routine basis to assess the level of function and concern about the problem; in others, the slightest deficit will be a major concern and they will bring up the subject themselves. Reversible, nonsurgical techniques such as intracavernous injection or vacuum tumescence devices should be used first, and may actually accelerate the spontaneous resolution of impotence and optimize the ultimate erectile quality. Some surgeons place penile prostheses at the time of the radical prostatectomy in men who are already impotent or who will not receive nerve-sparing prostatectomy, though this is not a widely accepted approach at this time. Instead, a delay of 6–12 months after prostatectomy is usually best before placement of a prosthesis, the longer period for patients who have had nerve-sparing prostatectomy to allow time for potential spontaneous resolution of impotence. Many men may want to delay any treatment even longer depending upon the pathologic diagnosis, their continence and psychological status, and their partners' attitudes.

Testosterone Replacement Therapy

Any patient with prostate cancer should not have testosterone replacement therapy initiated, because such therapy could exacerbate any existing tumor. A rare exception to this could be the patient who has confirmed hypogonadism, and has had a radical prostatectomy with no extraprostatic tumor on the pathologic examination, and no evidence of local or distant recurrence by exam, bone scan, and prostate specific antigen (PSA) 3 years after the surgery. Testosterone replacement can be achieved using intramuscular injection therapy or skin patches.

Oral Medication

Yohimbine and trazodone are now used for treatment of impotence. Success is rare with more severe organic impotence as after prostatectomy, but the drugs may be useful in patients who have a reduced libido as their primary complaint.

Vacuum Erection Devices

Externally applied vacuum suction devices induce penile tumescence and rigidity which are maintained with a constriction band at the base of the penis. This approach can be used by almost any patient with erectile dysfunction, with only mild short- or long-term risks.

Intracavernous Injection of Vasoactive Substances

Injection of vasoactive substances such as papaverine, phentolamine, and prostaglandin E_1 (PGE_1) has been successful in treatment of erectile impotence. Injection therapy is particularly effective in patients with neurogenic and mild to moderate vasculogenic impotence as after radical prostatectomy. Papaverine is no longer available for intracavernosal injection so PGE_1 is the only alternative for "off-label" use.

After prostatectomy, PGE_1 is administered in a test dose of 1–5 micrograms (μg); patients with concomitant vascular disease or diabetes will require test doses of 5–10 μg. Doses are increased up to about 20 μg until adequate response with some manual stimulation is achieved. Most patients with postprostatectomy impotence can achieve good function at doses of 5–10 μg. Since these doses are higher than those required for pure neurogenic impotence, it is likely that many prostatectomy patients have concomitant penile vascular deficits. Once a dose is selected, the patient is instructed on self-injection and given a prescription. The patient should be cautioned about the possibility of priapism and that an erection lasting more than 4 hr should be treated as an emergency. Such erections can be reversed by corporal aspiration and by intracavernous injection of α-adrenergic agents such as phenylephrine. Follow-up evaluations 1 to 3, 6, and 12 months later, and then annually will assess response, and possible complications such as penile pain, bruising, and penile fibrosis; if fibrosis occurs, therapy should stop. Research is ongoing to develop alternative methods of administering vasoactive agents, including intraurethral pellets or topical creams.

Penile Prostheses

Implantable penile prostheses are available in a range of models including malleable, articulated, and inflatable types. The simpler, noninflatable models are quicker to implant, have fewer mechanical problems and are cheaper than the inflatable models which offer the advantage of better concealment. Risks with any of the prostheses include infection, mechanical failure, and pain, but the frequency of these problems is relatively low and overall patient and partner acceptance is quite good.

Psychotherapy

Psychotherapy plays a role in the management of any patient's erectile dysfunction, starting with a presurgical discussion about the risks of surgically induced impotence, how a change of erectile function may affect him, and that a variety of treatment options are available should dysfunction develop. Adequate psychological support and counseling for the couple will improve the success of any therapy selected, and help overcome the anxiety, depression, and change in body image and control that accompany a diagnosis of cancer, repeated examinations, and surgery. Finally, a formal psychological consultation should be sought whenever the urologist or patient feels it is necessary.

CONCLUSIONS

There is a wide range of treatment options available for patients with incontinence or erectile dysfunction after radical prostatectomy. The patient should be presented with all of the appropriate options for therapy after an evaluation that is adequate to reach a clear diagnosis of the problem. Patient involvement in the decision process will result in the best clinical outcome and patient satisfaction level so that he can optimize his quality of life.

REFERENCES

1. Fowler FJ, Barry MJ, Lu-Yao G, et al: Patient-reported complications and follow-up treatment after radical prostatectomy. *Urology* 42:622–629, 1993.
2. Walsh PC, Partin AW, Epstein JI: Cancer control and quality of life following anatomical radical retropubic prostatectomy: results at 10 years. *J Urol* 152:1831–1836, 1994.
3. Lue TF: Impotence after prostatectomy. *Urol Clin North Am* 17:613–620, 1990.
4. Myers RP: Male urethral sphincteric anatomy and radical prostatectomy. *Urol Clin North Am* 18:211–227, 1991
5. Foote J, Yun S, Leach GE: Postprostatectomy incontinence. *Urol Clin North Am* 18:229–241, 1991.

6. Labasky RF: Urodynamics and evaluation of the incontinent patient. In Stein BS: *Clinical Urologic Practice*. New York, Norton, 1995, p 551.
7. Urinary Incontinence Guideline Panel. *Urinary Incontinence in Adults: Clinical Practice Guideline*. AHCPR Pub. No. 92-0038. Rockville, MD, Agency for Health Care Policy and Research, Public Health Service, U.S. Department of Health and Human Services. March 1992.
8. Labasky RF: Urodynamics. In Smith JA: *High Tech Urology*. Philadelphia, WB Saunders, 1992, p 144.
9. Sirls LT, Ganabathi K, Zimmern PE, et al: Management of urinary incontinence. In Stein BS: *Clinical Urologic Practice*. New York, Norton, 1995, pp 579–610.

13

Role of Cryosurgery in the Treatment of Localized Prostate Cancer

John A. Connolly
Katsuto Shinohara
Joseph C. Presti, Jr.
Peter R. Carroll

During 1994, 38,000 men died in the United States from prostate cancer and a further 200,000 men were newly diagnosed with this disease.[1] As mortality from prostate cancer climbs, medical debate continues over the optimal treatment for patients with localized disease, especially in terms of cure rates and treatment morbidity. Although there is no absolute consensus, most urologists agree that the treatment of choice for organ-confined prostate cancer (T1 and T2 tumors) is radical prostatectomy in younger, healthier patients.[2,3] Radiation therapy is an alternative treatment modality but questions have arisen regarding its efficiency. However, it is commonly offered to patients who are at higher surgical risk due to age, concurrent medical conditions or to patients who have locally advanced (T3) tumors.[4] Difficulty arises when choosing the best treatment for the older, but still healthy patient with localized disease, or for the younger patient with T3 disease or any patient with local recurrence following radiation therapy. The former form the bulk of newly diagnosed prostate cancer—over 50% of men are greater than 75 years old at first diagnosis and many patients, irrespective of age, have locally advanced disease at presentation.[5,6] These patients do poorly with conventional treatments (i.e., radical surgery and radiation therapy) in terms of both morbidity and cancer cure rates.[4,7,8]

A better treatment for localized prostate cancer which offers lower morbidity and better results in the long-term eradication of tumor is desirable for all patients, but especially for the categories outlined above where the benefits of conventional treatment are often outweighed by increased morbidity or poor cancer cure rates. Of the alternatives under investigation, cryosurgery is one of the more promising. This technique, which involves destruction of prostatic tissue by in situ freezing, is not new but has engendered renewed interest because of percutaneous probe placement and improvements in imaging and cryotechnology.[9-14] The goal of cryosurgery is to eradicate all cancer, while not damaging adjacent organs. If this goal can be reached, cryosurgery with localized tumors (T1/T2) should give cancer control results as good as radical prostatectomy. Locally advanced tumors that have not yet metastasized may be amenable to cryosurgical ablation more than conventional radical prostatectomy or radiation therapy, as the freezing zone can be advanced into the seminal vesicles or periprostatic tissue for destruction of extraprostatic cancer. An additional attraction of cryosurgery is the reported low morbidity, minimal blood loss, and the short hospital stay.

HISTORY OF CRYOSURGERY

Freezing as a treatment for cancer was first employed in the mid nineteenth century.[15] Early experiments with breast and gynecologic cancers showed reduction in tumor volumes and alleviation of pain, even with crude methods such as iced saline. Since its inception, cryosurgery has successfully been used in the treatment of melanomas, carcinoma of the skin, oral and ophthalmologic cancers, bronchial tumors, gastrointestinal cancers (especially esophageal, anorectal, and liver cancers) and genitourinary cancers, especially prostate and penile.[16]

In the 1960s and 1970s, cryosurgery of the prostate was carried out via the transurethral route as a treatment for both prostate cancer and benign prostatic hyperplasia.[17] Incomplete freezing and postoperative urinary retention were common. Attention focused for a time on alternative approaches to freezing the prostate, i.e., through an open perineal incision or through the suprapubic route, but despite use of thermal sensors and tactile sensation for monitoring, problems with adequate control of the freezing process persisted. This led to residual cancer in some patients and rectourethral or urethrocutaneous fistula formation in others.[18] Despite these limitations, open perineal cryosurgery had survival rates for all stages of disease equivalent to radical prostatectomy.[19] The technique, however, never became a widely accepted treatment for prostate cancer, mainly for reasons of morbidity.

In 1988, Onik described the ultrasound characteristics of the frozen prostate, and, in doing so, revitalized interest in this modality for treatment of localized prostate cancer.[20] He demonstrated that transrectal ultrasound (TRUS) could be used to monitor the freezing process to ensure adequate but not over treatment. TRUS could also help in accurate placement of the cryosurgical probes using the transperineal percutaneous route. More recently, the position of the ice-ball edge (visible as a hyperechoic rim on ultrasound) has been shown to correlate well with the extent of histologic damage in the dog prostate.[21] All of these developments have caused renewed interest in cryosurgery for treating localized prostate cancer which has gained momentum due to promising preliminary results, technical advances in cryosurgical instrumentation, and patient interest in new treatments that hold the promise of reduced morbidity.[12,13,22]

MECHANISMS OF CRYOSURGICAL TISSUE DESTRUCTION

For cell death to occur, actual freezing must take place. As the tissue temperature is progressively lowered, freezing first occurs in the extracellular compartment and microvascular network.[23] Formation of pure ice water in the extracellular compartment causes any remaining fluid in this compartment to be electrolyte rich and hyperosmolar. Free water is drawn from the intracellular compartment by the hyperosmolar extracellular environment, leading to protein denaturation and cell membrane damage. With continued lowering of the temperature, intracellular freezing becomes evident at −20° C and is complete at −40° C. Intracellular freezing causes cell destruction, and if it does not occur, the tissue cells may recover. Such recovery may take several months. With rapid freezing, the cells have less chance to lose their intracellular water and are therefore more susceptible to damage from intracellular ice crystal formation.[23]

Thawing is also a lethal process. As extracellular water melts, it is drawn into the intracellular compartment. Because the cell membranes have been damaged during freezing, they do not function normally and cell swelling and bursting occurs. During freezing and thawing, damage also occurs to the cells of the microvasculature, resulting in tissue anoxia. In vivo experiments on the canine prostate have shown that whole-gland tissue destruction is possible with cryosurgery resulting in coagulative necrosis of the gland.[20]

The cryoprobes currently in use (Accuprobe system) use liquid nitrogen (−196° C) as the coolant. The iceball is elliptical, approximately 4 cm in diameter and 4 cm in length along the probe.[12,14] Its size and temperature vary according to the percentage liquid nitrogen flow, e.g., at a flow of 100% the radius of the iceball is approximately 2 cm while a flow of 25% produces an iceball of approximately 1-cm radius.[12,14] The edge of the iceball, as seen on ultrasound, is 0° C and tissue 2–3 mm within the margin of the iceball is at a temperature of −20° C (a temperature which will produce tissue necrosis) at maximal liquid nitrogen flow.[12] At the part of the iceball furthest from the tip of the cryoprobe, this distance is probably 4–5 mm (Fig. 13.1). During a slow freeze, the distance from the

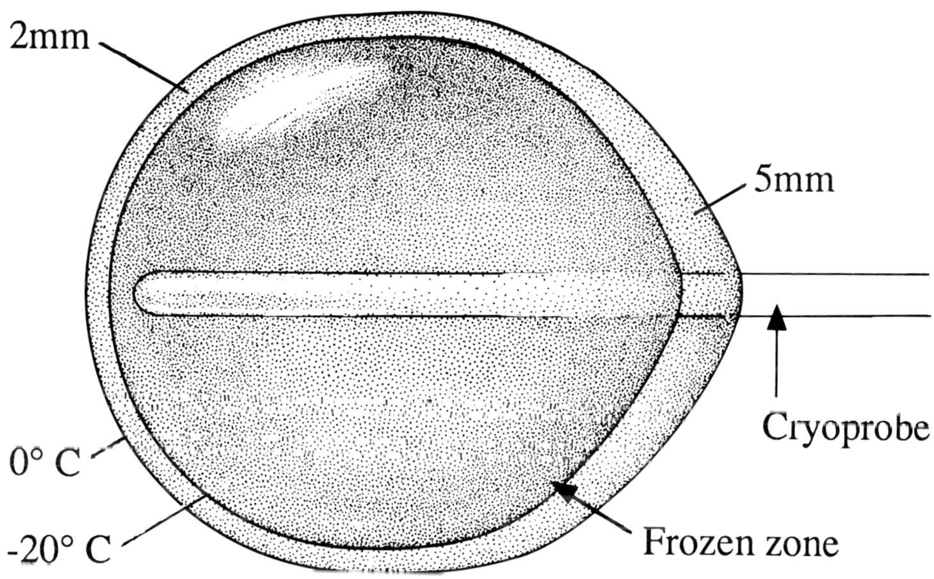

Fig. 13.1. The freeze zone or "iceball" measures approximately 4 cm in length at 100% flow of liquid nitrogen. A temperature of −20° C (i.e., low enough to cause cell death) exists 2 mm from the leading edge of the iceball near the tip of the cryoprobe, and 5 mm from the leading edge of the iceball furthest from the tip.

edge of the iceball (0° C) to the −20° C zone can be as much as 7 mm at the tip of the probe. This is due to slower liquid nitrogen flow with less efficient tissue freezing.

PATIENT SELECTION AND EVALUATION

In our practice, cryosurgery is offered to patients with localized prostate cancer who have a life expectancy, notwithstanding their tumor, of at least 10 years. The cryosurgical option is discussed with patients who are not good candidates for surgery, i.e., older patients and those with significant coexisting medical problems who have significant cancers, as well as patients with clinical T3 disease and patients who have local recurrence after radiation therapy. Our assumption (which at this time remains unproven) is that cryosurgery may be less morbid than radical prostatectomy in these patients while being more effective at eradicating cancer than radiation therapy. Our bias is to offer radical prostatectomy to younger men with clinically organ-confined disease. The lack of medium- and long-term follow-up with cryosurgery is emphasized to all patients.

Patients should have biopsy proven prostate cancer. Using both digital rectal examination (DRE) and transrectal ultrasound (TRUS), the size and location of prostatic tumors, seminal vesicle involvement, or extracapsular extension are noted. In addition to patients with visible tumors on ultrasound (T2, T3, and T4 lesions), patients with sonographically invisible lesions (T1c) are also considered for cryosurgery. Patients with suspected seminal vesicle involvement undergo seminal vesicle biopsy. Areas of gross extracapsular extension (ECE) are also biopsied.

Bone scans are done in accordance with current literature recommendations, with some modification (i.e., patients with a prostate specific antigen [PSA] of ≥ 10, Gleason score ≥ 7, and/or patients with known seminal vesicle involvement or gross extracapsular extension).[24] Pelvic lymph node dissection (PLND) is performed using the minilap technique in patients with PSA > 15 and Gleason sum ≥ 7, PSA > 25 and Gleason sum ≤ 6 or with gross T3 disease.[25,26] Serum PSA is obtained preoperatively in all patients. Acid phosphatase and computed tomography (CT) of the pelvis are not routinely carried out but are performed in patients at significant risk of pelvic lymph node metastases (i.e. $> 35\%$).[27] The rest of the preoperative workup is individualized for each patient but usually includes complete blood count (CBC), electrolytes, renal function tests, electrocardiograph, chest x-ray, type and screen, urinalysis, and urine culture. Patients with a positive urine culture are treated with a course of appropriate antibiotics prior to cryosurgery. We do not request autologous or donor directed blood.

Patients with locally extensive cancer or patients whose prostate glands are > 50 cc in size are placed on complete androgen blockade for at least 3 months prior to the cryosurgical procedure. The rationale of androgen deprivation is to shrink larger glands to a size that can be more easily treated with five cryoprobes (approximately 50 gm) and to reduce bulky extracapsular disease. The smaller prostate volume allows for tighter temperature gradients between the cryoprobes, thereby minimizing the likelihood of incomplete tissue freezing. Additionally, downsizing large prostates may widen the periprostatic space and help avoid inclusion of the pubic rami, pelvic muscles, and rectum in the freeze zone. Full staging (bone scan and pelvic lymph node dissection when indicated) is completed before starting antiandrogen treatment. Androgen deprivation therapy is discontinued after cryosurgery.

CRYOSURGICAL TECHNIQUE

Patients are admitted to hospital on the day of surgery and receive an enema bowel preparation and intravenous antibiotics prior to the procedure. After induction of anesthesia (general or regional), the patient is placed in the lithotomy position. The lower abdomen and perineum are shaved, prepared with betadine, and draped. If a pelvic lymph node dissection is indicated, it can be performed at a separate setting or under the same anesthetic. If the latter option is chosen, the node dissection should be carried out first and the nodes sent for frozen section analysis before cryotherapy is commenced.

A urethral catheter is passed and the bladder filled with normal saline. A suprapubic tube is placed under transrectal ultrasound guidance. A balloon filled with warm water is used around the tip of the transrectal ultrasound probe to improve image resolution and to help protect the rectal mucosa from freezing. A warming device is placed in the urethra after removing the Foley catheter, the purpose of which is to protect the urethra in the area of the voluntary sphincter, especially when freezing the apex of the gland, and also to protect the bladder neck. As there is no Food and Drug Administration (FDA) approved urethral warmer at this time, a device is constructed similar to that described by Cohen and Miller.[28] This device involves recirculating warmed saline (approximately 45° C) through a specially adapted double-lumen urethral catheter.

A multiprobe cryosurgical device (Accuprobe system, Cryomedical Sciences, Inc., Rockville, MD) is used for the freezing process. This recently developed cryosurgical system has five independently controllable delivery systems for liquid nitrogen that can be operated simultaneously.[22] The system has been designed to deliver liquid nitrogen to the tip of the probe in the most efficient manner possible, i.e., in a completely liquid state. This is achieved by subcooling the liquid nitrogen to −206° C and eliminating unwanted nitrogen gas through a vent system built into the probe. A problem with earlier cryoprobes was the formation of gas pockets at the probe tip leading to "choking" of flow as the vaporizing liquid nitrogen underwent rapid expansion. This resulted in further warming of the liquid nitrogen with more nitrogen gas formation and ultimately suboptimal temperatures at the probe tip. High pressure flow to the cryoprobe, insulation on the cryoprobe hose (polyethylene), and vacuum insulation of the cryoprobe itself help to keep the nitrogen in the liquid state. The insulated and ventilated probe (which measures 3.4 mm in diameter) provides efficient delivery of liquid nitrogen for tissue freezing while protecting the skin and subcutaneous tissues from exposure to the freezing liquid nitrogen.

Using a needle guide attached to the transrectal ultrasound probe, a diamond tip 18-gauge needle (Cook Urological, Spencer, Indiana) is placed transperineally into the prostate under ultrasound guidance. Five such needles are placed: two anterior and medially, two posterior and laterally, and one behind the urethra (Fig. 13.2). This distribution helps to ensure complete freezing of the prostate and they are placed in approximately the same arrangement regardless of tumor location. For a gland < 50 gm, the probes are placed approximately 1.2 cm from the anterior margin of the gland and equidistant from the proximal urethra, separated by approximately 1.8 cm. The posterior probes should also be placed about 1.2 cm from the posterior margin of the gland and 1.0 cm from the lateral aspects of the prostate. This ensures that lateral freezing is adequate before the iceball reaches the rectal wall. For optimal apical freezing, the anterior and posterior probes should angle medially to laterally from the apex to the base of the prostate. If the gland is

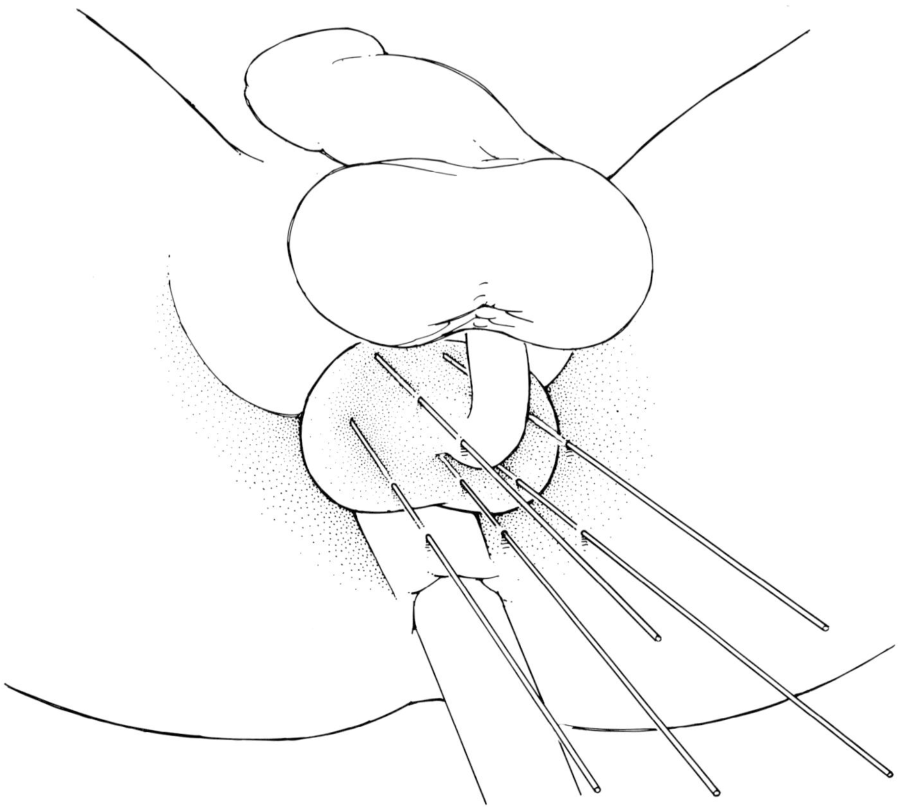

Fig. 13.2. With the patient in lithotomy position, the five needles are placed percutaneously into the prostate—two anteriorly, two posteriorly, and one below the urethra.

very large or if there is gross extension of tumor outside the capsule, use of a sixth probe may be necessary.

The needles are advanced cranially through the prostate until the proximal prostatic capsule is reached and needle position is checked with both transverse and longitudinal ultrasound views. If the seminal vesicles need to be treated, the posterior needles are advanced into the base of the organ. The inner core of each needle is withdrawn and a 0.038-inch J tipped wire (nontapered) advanced under ultrasound guidance until it emerges from the tip of the needle. The cannula is then carefully removed leaving the J-wire in position (Fig. 13.3). A fixed retraction device (we use the Buckwalter retractor) is set up above the operative site and used to fix the guidewires and prevent accidental dislodgement. A small incision (approximately ½ cm) is made in the skin at the exit point of each wire using a number 11 blade. A 12-French dilator is placed over each guidewire and advanced under ultrasound guidance to the base of the prostate. A 12-French hollow sheath is then passed over each dilator and the dilator removed. The location of the tip of the sheath is carefully checked by ultrasound after injecting saline into the cannula to better visualize it (Fig. 13.4). A cryoprobe is placed through each cannula and the cannula pulled back to expose the tip of the cryoprobe to the prostatic tissue. After a final ultra-

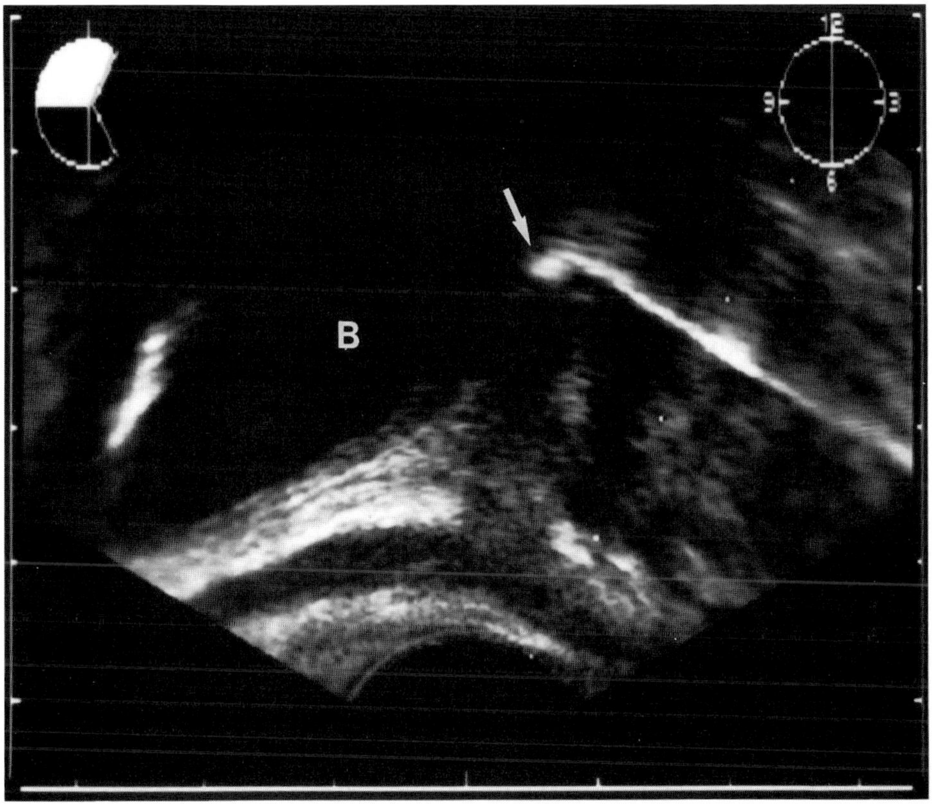

Fig. 13.3. Longitudinal ultrasound image showing a J-tip guidewire in correct position with the tip of the guidewire (*arrow*) at the proximal prostatic capsule, adjacent to the bladder (*B*).

sound check of probe position, liquid nitrogen flow is started. The probe tip temperature is initially lowered to −70° C to "stick" the tip of the probe to the prostate tissue. This, along with support from the fixed retractor, ensures that the probes do not move from their correct positions.

Freezing is commenced using the anterior probes first. When anterior freezing is of adequate size, freezing with the posterior probes is started. The iceball is monitored on TRUS where the edge is seen as a densely hyperechoic rim. Freezing is continued laterally beyond the prostatic capsule for a distance of 3–4 mm. In areas of ECE, the iceball is allowed to grow until it is beyond the tumor area. Posteriorly, the rim of the freeze zone is allowed to pass through the prostate capsule and into the muscularis propria of the rectum, but no deeper than this (Fig. 13.5). This allows adequate freezing of the posterior aspect of the prostate but does not damage the rectal wall, the thickest part of which is the mucosa which also has the best blood supply. Additional rectal protection may be achieved by placing warmed water in the transrectal probe balloon during the posterior freezing process and changing this water frequently. Lee and associates describe a method whereby 18-gauge introducer needles are used as crude thermosensors to evaluate the effectiveness of the iceball.[12] Needles are placed under ultrasound guidance at the

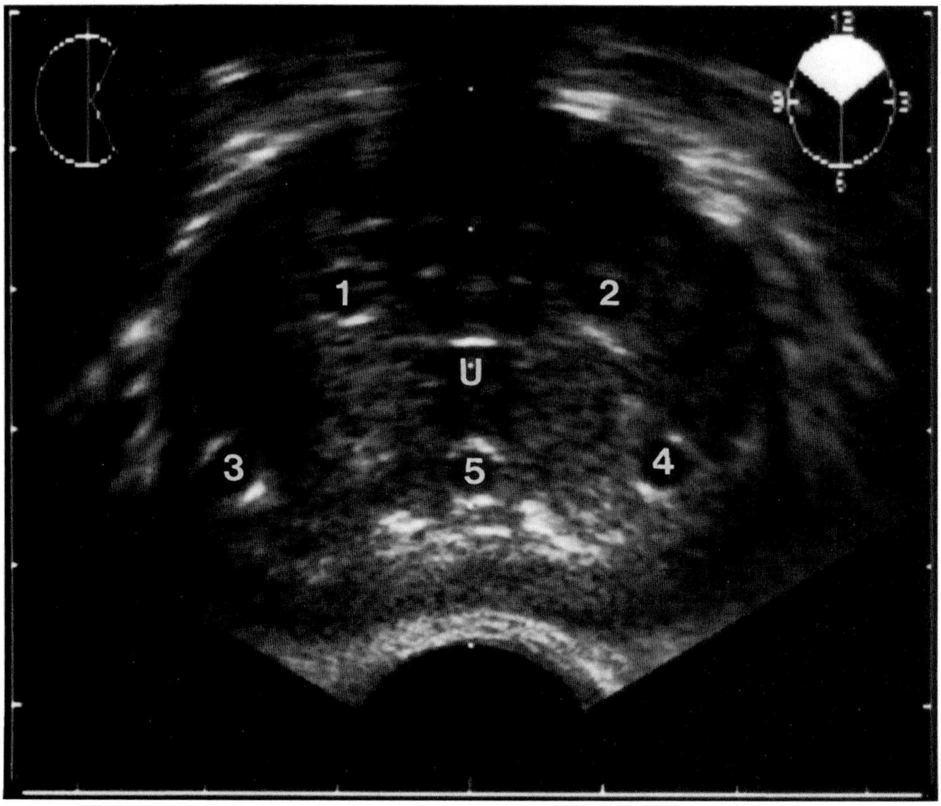

Fig. 13.4. Transverse ultrasound image showing position of the five sheaths (1–5) before insertion of the cryoprobes. The urethra (*U*) contains the urethral warmer.

anterior, posterior, and apical margins of the prostate. When the temperature is approximately −20° C, the needle becomes fixed to the iceball and cannot be retracted. When available, sensors that provide an actual temperature readout can be used at these locations.

After the first freezing cycle is completed, the prostate is thawed. As the iceball recedes, the prostate once again becomes visible on TRUS. We now routinely perform a second freeze/thaw cycle in all patients. The second freeze cycle is started as soon as the periphery of the prostate is revisualized. The probes are kept in their original position. If the iceball does not adequately extend to the apex of the prostate, the cryoprobes are pulled into the apex and a third freeze/thaw cycle carried out (Fig. 13.6). To calculate the distance the probes should be withdrawn, we measure the distance from the edge of the iceball to the apex of the prostate and add 8 mm. The 8-mm addition overcompensates for the 5-mm zone at the posterior edge of the iceball that will have temperatures between 0° C and −20° C (levels which are probably inadequate for cell death). Although the iceball is allowed to extend into the levators, care should be taken not to freeze beyond the prostatic apex more than a few millimeters as the voluntary sphincter may be damaged. If the remaining apical tissue is relatively large in size, a fourth freeze/thaw cycle is added

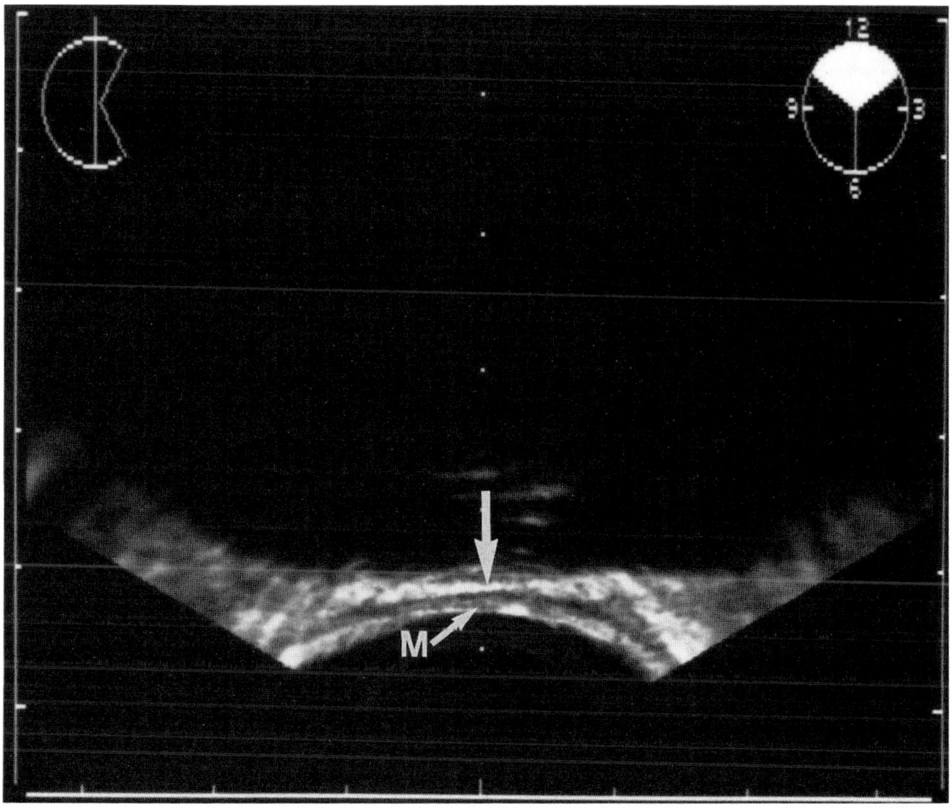

Fig. 13.5. Transverse ultrasound image showing the edge of the iceball touching the muscularis propria of the rectum (*arrow*). This is the furthest the iceball should be allowed to advance. The thick rectal mucosa (*M*) is seen below the edge of the freeze zone.

at the apex. Following the final thawing process, the cryoprobes and urethral warming device are removed. The perineal incisions are closed with an absorbable suture. A Foley catheter is placed and the patient returns to the recovery room with continuous bladder irrigation running through the suprapubic tube. Although this is our standard practice, the degree of hematuria is usually very minor. The Foley catheter is removed the following morning and the suprapubic tube is removed in most patients at 2 weeks after surgery. Before removal the patient must demonstrate an adequate flow rate with a low postvoid residual.

A PSA is checked at 3 months postoperatively and patients undergo TRUS and biopsy at 6 months, along with PSA measurements at that time. At the postoperative TRUS, biopsies are taken from the apex, mid region, base, lateral prostatic edge, base of the seminal vesicle, and from any other area suspicious for residual cancer. Biopsy specimens are taken under ultrasound guidance using an 18-gauge needle loaded on a spring action automatic biopsy device. In our practice, biopsies showing no evidence of prostate cancer are considered negative. Patients who demonstrate viable acinar tissue on biopsy and where the PSA is undetectable or stable are considered to have no evidence of disease

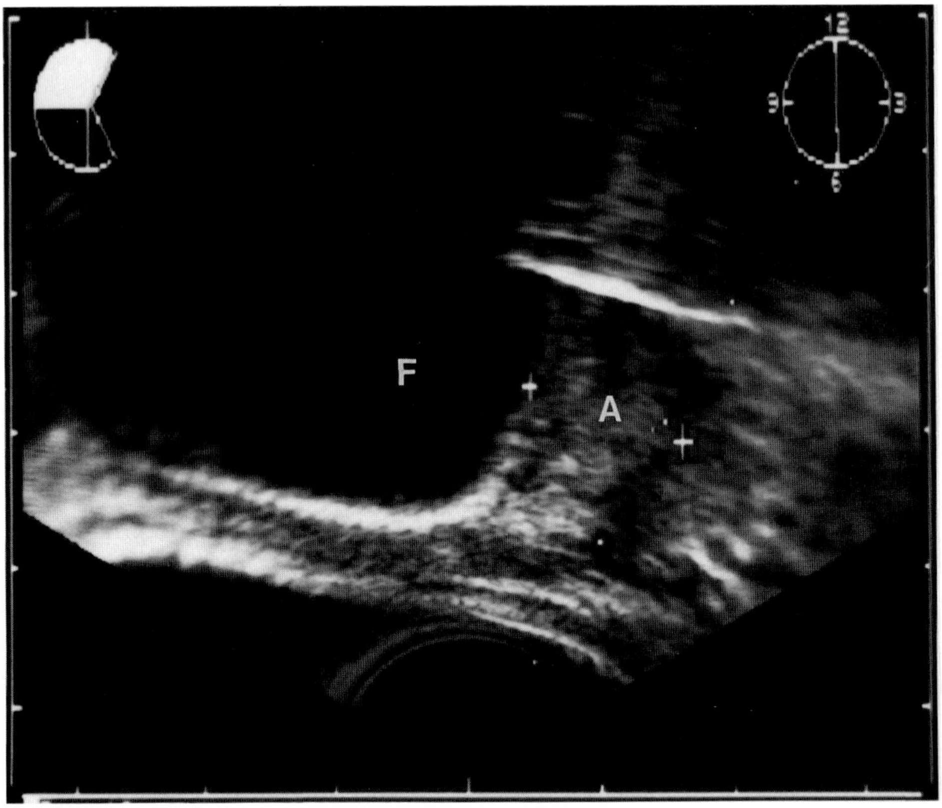

Fig. 13.6. Longitudinal ultrasound image showing freeze zone (*F*) and residual apical tissue (*A*).

(NED). Patients who develop a rising PSA after cryosurgery and who have negative biopsies undergo additional imaging to assess for metastatic disease. If biopsies are positive for cancer and there is no evidence of metastatic disease, repeat cryosurgery, radiation therapy, salvage prostatectomy, or androgen deprivation are offered to patients.

RESULTS OF CRYOSURGERY

Initial results with cryosurgery of the prostate have been encouraging. Onik demonstrated a 6.7% positive biopsy rate at 3 months after cryosurgery in 15 patients.[9] The post-cryosurgery PSAs in these 15 patients ranged, however, from 0 to 9.8 ng/ml (mean 1.5 ± 2.6 ng/ml). Only 3 of 15 patients (20%) had an undetectable PSA (< 0.1 ng/ml) at 3 months after cryosurgery. Complications described by Onik included freezing of the rectum in 5.9%, rectourethral fistula in 2.9%, and sloughing of prostatic urethral tissue in 4.4%. Sixty-five percent of patients were impotent after the procedure. Other complications included perineal ecchymosis, penile edema, and ileus (percent rates not published).

Bahn and associates described persistent cancer in 7.7% and 2.3% of patients at 3 months (130 patients) and 12 months (43 patients) respectively.[13] It is unclear how many of their patients had benign epithelial elements seen in their postcryosurgical biopsies. In

TABLE 13.1. Prostate Cancer Stage in Patients Undergoing Cryoablation

Stage	*Number of Patients* (%)*
T1c	11 (11)
T2	33 (31)
T3a/b	32 (30)
T3c	26 (25)
T4	3 (3)

*Does not include two patients who underwent cryosurgery for local recurrence following radical prostatectomy.

their report, a PSA value of > 1.0 ng/ml at 3 months after cryosurgery was 70% sensitive for cancer and 88% specific. Complications included a rectourethral fistula rate of 2.4% (80% of these were in patients who previously had radiation therapy), severe outlet obstruction in 2.9%, total incontinence in 2.3%, stress incontinence in 6.2%, pelvic pain/dysuria in 1.5%, impotence at 1 year in 41% of previously potent men, and a TURP was necessary in 1% of patients. Mean PSA values at 3 months were 1.4 ± 8.1 ng/ml and at 12 months were 1.2 ± 5.0 ng/ml. They did not indicate the number of patients with an undetectable PSA after cryosurgery.

At the University of California, San Francisco, 102 patients have undergone 107 cryosurgical procedures between July 1993 and February 1995. Their ages ranged from 50 to 70 years old with a mean age of 68 years. Forty-four patients had cancer which appeared to be confined within the prostatic capsule on transrectal ultrasound (T1 and T2 lesions). The remaining patients had more extensive disease by TRUS (Table 13.1). Ten patients had previously been treated with radiation therapy to the prostate, 58 patients had preoperative neoadjuvant hormone deprivation, and eight patients had cryosurgery carried out in our unit after failed cryosurgery elsewhere. Mean hospital stay was 2.3 days and mean length of suprapubic drainage was 11.3 days. Forty-five pelvic lymph node dissections were carried out (using the indications already described).

Seventy-six patients in our series have PSA follow-up of ≥ 3 months, and of these 38 (50%) have a PSA < 0.1 ng/dl, 21 (28%) have a PSA in the 0.1–0.5 ng/dl range, and 17 (22%) have a PSA of ≥ 0.5 ng/dl. Residual cancer was seen at 6 months after cryosurgery in 24% of patients and residual benign glands in 73%. When our results are analyzed over time, it is evident that there is a learning curve for cryosurgery (Table 13.2). With increased experience and improvements in technique (i.e., routine double freezing, periprostatic tissue freezing, and careful apical freezing) the rates of detectable PSA, positive biopsies, and residual benign glands have all fallen.

TABLE 13.2. Cryosurgical Results

Case No.	*Detectable PSA*	*Residual Glands*	*Positive Biopsy*
1–30	25/30 (83%)	22/25* (88%)	12/27 (44%)
31–107	22/58 (38%)	16/27† (59%)	2/31 (6%)

*Status unknown in two patients.
†Status unknown in four patients.

TABLE 13.3. Complications of Cryosurgery

Obstruction requiring transurethral resection	25/107 (23%)
Penile numbness	11/107 (10%)
Incontinence	4/107 (4%)
Epididymitis	4/107 (4%)
Prolonged perineal pain	3/107 (3%)
Osteitis pubis	2/107 (2%)
Rectourethral fistula	1/107 (1%)

Our experience with cryosurgical complications is outlined in Table 13.3. Obstruction requiring TURP was required in 23% of patients, usually 2–3 months postoperatively and usually preceded by urinary tract infection. Between July 1993 and May 1994, the need for postcryosurgical TURP was 17% but this figure increased to 44% between June 1994 and December 1994, coincident with the introduction of a different urethral warming device and with a policy of more aggressive freezing. Ten percent of patients complained of penile numbness of varying extent and duration after the procedure. Rectourethral fistula was rare, occurring in one patient who had failed radiation therapy prior to cryosurgery.

DISCUSSION

A resurgence of interest in cryosurgery as a treatment for localized prostate cancer has occurred over the past 4–5 years. Disaffection with radical prostatectomy and radiation therapy cure rates (especially in patients with local extension of cancer into the tissues or seminal vesicles) and the perception of relatively high morbidity with these treatments have been the impetus behind the search for alternatives. Although operative mortality is low (ranging from 0% to 0.7%),[2,5] it remains an important factor in the overall assessment of radical prostatectomy. Radical surgery may have significant morbidity. Pulmonary embolus, deep venous thrombosis, and myocardial infarction are relatively rare (0.7%, 1.1%, and 0.4% respectively) but other complications are more common.[2] Rectal injury has been reported in 1–11% of patients,[29,30] rates of urinary incontinence vary from 0.8% to 42% (depending on the definitions employed),[2,5] impotence occurs in 32% to 89% of men,[3,7] and blood transfusion is required in 5% to 100% of men.[2,31] As for cancer control, positive margins at the time of radical prostatectomy (associated with high rates of local recurrence and PSA failure) range from 4.3% to 46%.[32,33] Metastases, local recurrence, or a detectable PSA alone after radical prostatectomy have been reported in up to 52% of patients at 10 years.[2]

Radiation therapy, also, is not without significant morbidity. In one large series, complications included radiation proctitis (5.4%), cystitis (5.1%), urethral stricture (5.4%), and impotence (30–61%).[34] Pulmonary embolus and lymphocele formation, though rare, sometimes occur. Of great concern are reports of high positive biopsy rates following radiation therapy (80–90% after 5 years) and more aggressive tumors (as evidenced by PSA doubling times and histologic dedifferentiation) in patients after radiation.[35,36]

Especially in patients with T3 disease, radical prostatectomy, radiation therapy, and hormone therapy all have limited long-term efficacy in eradication of cancer. It has been argued that careful patient selection and greater attention to the technical aspects of radical prostatectomy would improve complication rates and positive margin rates in patients with localized disease, but this remains to be proven.[36]

Recent cryosurgical reports have emphasized the potential for curing localized prostate cancer with less morbidity than radical prostatectomy.[9,13] The use of transrectal ultrasound imaging, percutaneous techniques, and new cryotechnology have transformed cryosurgery from a poorly controlled, morbid operation to a minimally invasive procedure with accurate freezing and fewer side effects. Results to date indicate that, in the short term at least, cryosurgery may cure localized prostate cancer.[9,13] At 6 months, our negative biopsy rate (no cancer) was 76%, while the number of patients with an undetectable PSA was 47%. Overall, 73% of our patients had some benign epithelial elements seen on postcryosurgical biopsy, and the true meaning of this is not yet known. Onik reports a 3-month negative biopsy rate of 93.3% in 15 patients but this excellent cancer-free rate is balanced by an undetectable PSA rate of just 20%. Longer follow-up is necessary to confirm cure in patients with early negative biopsies and to elucidate the parameters that will define cryosurgical success. In one study with long-term follow-up, Bonney and colleagues reported 5-year survival for patients undergoing open perineal cryosurgery as equivalent to radical prostatectomy. This study did not address rates of recurrent or residual tumor and the use of androgen deprivation therapy in some patients renders their results difficult to interpret.[37]

It is our view that negative biopsies and an undetectable PSA must be demonstrated at 6 months and at 1 year following cryosurgery if the patient is to be considered "cured." Continuing hormone therapy after cryosurgery may lead to false negative biopsies and falsely low PSA values. Even if biopsies do not show cancer, residual acinar tissue implies incomplete destruction of the prostate. This scenario is likely to be associated with cancer recurrence as the quality and/or extent of the freezing process has been inadequate. Similarly, a detectable PSA postoperatively, even with biopsies that show only scar tissue, raises the question of future clinical recurrence of prostate cancer.

Although cryosurgery is relatively noninvasive, we have encountered significant morbidity in our own patients: approximately 23% required transurethral resection of the prostate (TURP) to eliminate obstructive, necrotic prostatic tissue from the prostatic fossa or to remove free-floating necrotic prostate from the bladder; incontinence occurred in 4% (15% when 12 patients who developed stress urinary incontinence after TURP are considered) and impotence in 84%. Many of the patients (46%) who required TURP had significant initial problems with continence despite conservative resection. Recent higher rates of urinary retention and incontinence have also been noted by others and may be due to more aggressive freezing of the prostate in an attempt to eliminate all prostatic tissue.[14,38] From mid-1994, our TURP rate in cryosurgical patients increased, coincident both with FDA denying approval of an investigational urethral warming device and the use of multiple freeze/thaw cycles. Although we have since used a "home-made" warming device, this may not adequately protect the bladder neck and voluntary sphincter areas. More effective urethral warming and use of thermosensors to establish adequate freezing and help protect other structures might reduce the incidence of urinary retention and improve incontinence rates. However, tissue sloughing and the need to surgically remove this tissue in some patients may be inevitable if negative biopsies and an undetectable PSA are to be achieved.

Cryosurgery is a flexible treatment modality and can be repeated in patients with residual or recurrent cancer. We have carried out recryoablation in eight patients with no added morbidity. Treatment of local recurrences after radical retropubic prostatectomy (RRP) or radiation therapy (RT) is also possible. In our experience, one of two patients who had cryosurgery for local recurrence after RRP had an undetectable PSA and no incontinence with more than 6 months follow-up. Previous radiation treatment does not exclude use of cryosurgery, but is associated with an increased rate of complications. A recent report from the University of Chicago quotes a 44% incontinence rate in these patients and Bahn and colleagues state that 80% of their rectourethral fistulas occurred in patients who had been previously irradiated.[13,39] Cryosurgery as initial treatment does not exclude other treatments (radiation therapy or androgen deprivation) at a later date should they become necessary. Performing a radical prostatectomy, however, in a patient who has already had cryosurgery might be associated with an increased risk of rectal injury. The iceball is routinely propagated through the muscularis propria of the rectum and this may result in scarring and adhesion of the prostate to the rectum. Although experience with salvage prostatectomy following failed cryosurgery is very limited, a recent report of six cases describes no rectal injury in any patient and an undetectable PSA after surgery in five patients.[40]

The rate of early impotence in all series is high, but seems to improve with time. In one report, 90% of patients were impotent at 6 months but by one year this had fallen to 41%.[13] Early postcryosurgical impotence is likely due to a deliberate policy of allowing the iceball to extend into the lateral periprostatic tissue which contains the neurovascular bundles. In our view, this is an important technical point if all prostatic tissue is to be destroyed. In addition, many patients are on androgen ablation therapy for several months prior to cryosurgery and this may contribute to initial postoperative impotence. Penile numbness was a problem in 10% of our patients but proved transient in the majority, lasting only a few months. This may be due to freezing of branches of the pudendal nerves during apical prostatic freezing.

To date, the overall costs of cryosurgery are not significantly different from radical prostatectomy or radiation therapy. This reflects the relatively high cost of disposables with this procedure as most patients stay in hospital overnight only. At our institution, the average cost and charges for cryosurgery are approximately 80–85% of those for radical prostatectomy. These costs do not, however, take into account expenditure on treating complications.

In order to accurately assess the role for cryosurgery in the treatment of localized prostate cancer, considerable research is still needed. The amount of freeze/thaw cycles necessary, the optimal freezing temperature for prostatic tissue, the use of thermocouples to confirm adequate freezing and to protect the bladder neck, the voluntary sphincter, and the rectum all need further research. Cryosurgical technology is also still in the development stages. The Accuprobe system represents a great advance for delivery of liquid nitrogen to the prostate, but an adequate urethral warming device has yet to be developed and approved by the FDA. Ultimately, the test of cryosurgery will be a prospective controlled trial, comparing it with other treatment modalities, e.g., RRP/RT/watchful waiting. Until cryosurgical technology is fully refined, however, a comparative study between it and radical prostatectomy might be premature. It should be noted also that cryosurgery is not technically easy, has a significant learning curve, and is best carried out by those with extensive TRUS experience.

SUMMARY

Cryosurgery is one option for the management of prostate cancer. It is associated with limited, though significant, morbidity and it may be repeated should recurrence of disease be noted. Although early results appear promising, the long-term results of the procedure are unknown and patients need to be advised of this. Follow-up is too short to recommend this procedure to the young, healthy man with localized disease as an equivalent option to radical prostatectomy. The morbidity and efficacy of the procedure need to be validated in prospective and controlled trials. Suitable endpoints for analysis would be short and long-term complication rates (including erectile function, incontinence rates, and the need for other procedures, e.g., TURP), as well as postcryosurgical PSA concentrations and early and delayed ultrasound-guided biopsy results. Also, the impact of cryosurgery on the morbidity and efficacy of subsequent radical prostatectomy has not been determined as yet. In our hands, cryosurgery of the prostate is still a procedure undergoing frequent modifications in technique as we gain experience and make changes in technique. The most significant development to date has been the use of multiple freeze/thaw cycles and freezing of the periprostatic tissue. This has resulted in better rates of PSA undetectability and negative post-treatment biopsies. Development of a better urethral warming device and use of thermosensors to control more precisely the freezing process are anticipated future developments that may lower morbidity and improve cancer-free rates.

REFERENCES

1. Boring CC, Squires TS, Tong T, et al: Cancer statistics, 1994. *CA Cancer J Clin* 44:7, 1994.
2. Zincke H, Oesterling JE, Blute ML, et al: Long-term (15 years) results after radical prostatectomy for clinically localized (stage T2c or lower) prostate cancer. *J Urol* 152:1850, 1994.
3. Walsh PC, Partin AW, Epstein JI: Cancer control and quality of life following anatomical radical retropubic prostatectomy: results at 10 years. *J Urol* 152:1831, 1994.
4. Kabalin JN, Hodge KK, McNeal JE, et al: Identification of residual cancer in the prostate following radiation therapy: role of transrectal ultrasound guided biopsy and prostate specific antigen. *J Urol* 142:326, 1989.
5. Murphy GP, Mettlin C, Menck H, et al: National patterns of prostate cancer treatment by radical prostatectomy: results of a survey by the American College of Surgeons Commission on Cancer. *J Urol* 152:1817, 1994.
6. Scardino PT: Early detection of prostate cancer. *Urol Clin North Am* 16:635, 1989.
7. Fowler FJ Jr, Barry MJ, Lu-Yao G, et al: Patient-reported complications and follow-up treatment after radical prostatectomy. The national medicare experience: 1988–1990. *Urology* 42:622, 1993.
8. Epstein JI, Pizov G, Walsh PC: Correlation of pathologic findings with progression after radical retropubic prostatectomy. *CA* 71:3582, 1993.
9. Onik GM, Cohen JK, Reyes GD, et al: Transrectal ultrasound-guided percutaneous radical cryosurgical ablation of the prostate. *CA* 72:1291, 1993
10. Chodak GW: Cryosurgery of the prostate revisited. *CA* 72:1145, 1993.
11. Miller RJ, Cohen JK, Merlotti LA: Percutaneous transperineal cryosurgical ablation of the

prostate for the primary treatment of clinical stage C adenocarcinoma of the prostate. *Urology* 44:170, 1994.

12. Lee F, Bahn DK, McHugh TA, et al: US-guided percutaneous cryoablation of prostate cancer. *Radiology* 192:769, 1994.
13. Bahn DK, Lee F, Solomon MH, et al: Prostate cancer: US-guided percutaneous cryoablation. *Radiology* 194:551, 1995.
14. Zippe CD: Cryosurgical ablation for prostate cancer: a current review. *Semin Urol* 13(2):148, 1995.
15. Bird HM: James Arnott, M.D. (Aberdeen) 1797–1883: a pioneer in refrigeration analgesia. *Anesthesia* 4:10, 1949.
16. Gage AA: Cryosurgery in the treatment of cancer. *Surg Gynecol Obstet* 174:73, 1992.
17. Gonder M, Soanes W, Shulman S: Cryosurgical treatment of the prostate. *Invest Urol* 3:372, 1966.
18. O'Donoghue EPN, Milleman L, Flocks R, et al: Cryosurgery for carcinoma of the prostate. *Urology* 5:308, 1975.
19. Loening S, Lubaroff D: Cryosurgery and immunotherapy for prostatic cancer. *Urol Clin North Am* 11:327, 1984.
20. Onik G, Cobb C, Cohen J, et al: US characteristics of frozen prostate. *Radiology* 168:629, 1988.
21. Littrup PJ, Montie J, Mody A, et al: Prostatic cryotherapy: ultrasonographic and pathological correlation in the canine model. *Urology* 44:175, 1994.
22. Chang Z, Finkelstein JJ, Ma H, et al: Development of a high-performance multiprobe cryosurgical device. *Biomed Instrument Technol* 28:383, 1994.
23. Baust JG, Chang ZH: Cryosurgery: underlying mechanisms of damage. Presented at the Second Annual Meeting of the Society of Urologic Cryosurgery, Dallas, TX, October 8–9, 1994.
24. Oesterling JE: Using PSA to eliminate the staging radio nuclide bone scan. Significant economic implications. *Urol Clin North Am* 20(4):705, 1993.
25. Wolf JS Jr, Shinohara K, Kerlikowske KM, et al: Selection of patients for laparoscopic pelvic lymphadenectomy prior to radical prostatectomy: a decision analysis. *Urology* 42:680, 1993.
26. Narayan P, Fournier G, Gajendran V, et al: Utility of preoperative serum prostate-specific antigen concentration and biopsy Gleason score in predicting risk of pelvic lymph node metastases in prostate cancer. *Urology* 44:519, 1994.
27. Wolf JS Jr, Cher M, Dall'era M, et al: The use and accuracy of cross-sectional imaging and fine needle aspiration cytology for detection of pelvic lymph node metastases before radical prostatectomy. *J Urol* 153:993, 1995.
28. Cohen JK, Miller RP: Thermal protection of urethra during cryosurgery of prostate. *Cryobiology* 31:313, 1994.
29. Borland RN, Walsh PC: The management of rectal injury during radical retropubic prostatectomy. *J Urol* 147:905, 1992.
30. Lassen PM, Kearse WS Jr: Rectal injuries during radical perineal prostatectomy. *Urology* 45:266, 1995.
31. Haab F, Boccon-Gibod L, Delmas V, et al: Perineal versus retropubic radical prostatectomy for T1, T2 prostate cancer. *Br J Urol* 74:626, 1994.
32. Jones EC: Resection margin status in radical retropubic prostatectomy specimens: relationship to type of operation, tumor size, tumor grade and local tumor extension. *J Urol* 144:89, 1990.

33. Morton RA, Steiner MS, Walsh PC: Cancer control following anatomical radical prostatectomy: an interim report. *J Urol* 145:1197, 1991.

34. Shipley WU, Zietman AL, Hanks GE, et al: Treatment related sequelae following external beam radiation for prostate cancer: a review with an update in patients with stages T1 and T2 tumor. *J Urol* 152:1799, 1994.

35. Stamey TA, Ferrari MK, Schmid HP: The value of serial prostate specific antigen determinations 5 years after radiotherapy: steeply increasing values characterize 80% of patients. *J Urol* 150:1856, 1993.

36. Walsh PC: Editorial: the status of radical prostatectomy in the United States in 1993: where do we go from here? *J Urol* 152:1816, 1994.

37. Bonney WW, Platz CE, Fallon B, et al: Cryosurgery in prostatic cancer: survival. *Urology* 19:37, 1982.

38. Cox RL, Crawford ED: Complications of cryosurgical ablation of the prostate to treat localized adenocarcinoma of the prostate. *Urology* 45:932, 1995.

39. Bales GT, Williams M, Chodak GW: Initial outcomes with cryosurgery in prostate cancer patients having failed radiation therapy. *J Urol* 151:436A, 1994.

40. Grampsas SA, Miller GJ, Crawford ED: Salvage radical prostatectomy after failed transperineal cryotherapy: histologic findings from prostate whole-mount specimens correlated with intraoperative transrectal ultrasound images. *Urology* 45:936, 1995.

INDEX